Take Control of Your Health

THE ESSENTIAL ROADMAP TO
MAKING THE RIGHT HEALTH CARE DECISIONS

Take Control
of Your Health

WILLIAM FELDMAN, MD, FRCPC

Professor Emeritus of Pediatrics and Public Health Sciences
University of Toronto

KEY PORTER BOOKS

Library and Archives Canada Cataloguing in Publication

Feldman, William
Take control of your health : the essential roadmap to making the right health
care decisions / William Feldman.

Includes index.
ISBN 978-1-55263-880-4

1. Patient participation—Canada. 2. Medical personnel and patient—Canada.
3. Evidence-based medicine—Canada. 4. Medical care—Canada. I. Title.

R727.42.F45 2007   610.69'6   C2006-905964-0

The publisher gratefully acknowledges the support of the Canada Council for the Arts and
the Ontario Arts Council for its publishing program. We acknowledge the support of the
Government of Ontario through the Ontario Media Development Corporation's Ontario
Book Initiative.

We acknowledge the financial support of the Government of Canada through the Book
Publishing Industry Development Program (BPIDP) for our publishing activities.

Key Porter Books Limited
Six Adelaide Street East, Tenth Floor
Toronto, Ontario
Canada M5C 1H6

www.keyporter.com

Text design: Martin Gould
Electronic formatting: Jean Lightfoot Peters

Printed and bound in Canada

07 08 09 10 11 5 4 3 2 1

Acknowledgements

I would like to thank Brian Feldman, Mark Feldman, Leonard Feldman, Adelle Atkinson, Rick Salutin, Paula Chabanais, Genevieve Rebello, Jess Rogers, and Kelly Lang for their help.

Table of Contents

Foreword

In writing this book, I have two objectives. The first is to attempt to explain why more and more patients are seeking alternative health care. The second is to explain the meaning and importance of evidence-based medicine. It is my hope and belief that when patients know how to ask the right questions of their health care providers, they will be better equipped to make appropriate decisions. Some patients will wish to go even further, and they may want to look at the answers for themselves. This book should provide patients with the knowledge and skills required to evaluate whether any recommended health intervention—from preventing an illness to treating it—will do more good than harm.

In the chapters on prevention, screening, diagnosis, prognosis, treatment, and clinical practice guidelines, case scenarios from the real world are used. These scenarios are intended to be used as examples only and are not meant to replace a visit to your doctor or alternative care provider. In these examples, brief stories describing clinical health issues are used to show how patients and family members can acquire and evaluate the evidence necessary to make decisions, from minor—should I give my child medication for his cold?—to major—should I have a mastectomy for my breast cancer?

CHAPTER 1

The Importance/Role of Evidence-Based Medicine

The recent information that a widely prescribed medication for arthritis, Vioxx, is more dangerous than much
less expensive and equally effective drugs has made the
public very anxious. Whom can you trust when making
decisions about your health care?

There have recently been a number of other widely
reported anxiety-provoking news items: autism is
thought to be caused by certain immunizations; kidney
problems are due to a cholesterol-lowering medication;
suicidal tendencies develop in teenagers taking antidepressants; the list goes on.

Centuries ago, illness was believed to be due to bad
spirits, witchcraft, the devil, or the wishes of our enemies. In some parts of the world these ideas are still
widely held. Even in the developed world, pilgrimages
to Lourdes are still undertaken to rid sick people of evil
spirits. The task of the physician was to help patients
cope with serious chronic and life-threatening diseases
and to provide various medicines and procedures such

as using bloodsucking leeches to remove evil spirits. Because most illnesses were short-lived, especially the most common ones caused by viruses, the therapy provided by the physician was believed to have helped the patient. The patient usually got rid of the virus with the help of his/her own immune system, however. Naturally, the provider of the treatment was revered and believed to have god-like qualities—who else can remove bad spirits?

For many hundreds of years, physicians studied and learned more about the anatomy of the human body and how the different body systems worked. During the last two hundred years, doctors have learned that numerous illnesses are caused by bacteria, many of which can be found in our food and drinking water. Public health measures to guarantee clean foods and water have had a major impact on our health. For example, in England and Wales from the mid-nineteenth century to the beginning of the twentieth century there was a dramatic decrease in mortality, ninety-two per cent of which was caused by a decline in deaths due to infections. This striking decrease occurred long before antibiotics were discovered and was associated largely with the purification of drinking water and more hygienic methods of sewage disposal. Commercial pasteurization and bottling of milk were introduced in the late nineteenth century, and by the beginning of the twentieth century deaths due to non-respiratory tuberculosis in children had dropped sharply.[1]

Immunizations, antibiotics and, more recently, antiviral medications have further led to much longer and healthier lives. Newer technologies, such as various laboratory and x-ray procedures, improvements in surgical techniques, as well as anti-cancer medicines and genetic tests have all had a tremendous impact not only on our health and longevity but also on our quality of life.

And yet, even though physicians in their research and practices have largely been responsible for producing many of these remarkable changes, the faith the public once had in doctors appears to have diminished. In 1975, Ivan Illich published a widely read book called *Medical Nemesis*, in which he wrote "...the medical establishment has become a major threat to health."[2] According to a prominent British doctor, Lord Turnberg, "it seems that trust in doctors is inversely related to the scientific basis of our practice. We were accorded most authority when we least deserved it."

In other words, in an era in which physicians really do have the knowledge and skills necessary to help millions, some patients are turning away from the medical profession in favour of alternative health practitioners. Complementary and alternative medicine (CAM)—practised by homeopaths, naturopaths, herbalists, etc.—is now used by over forty per cent of the U.S. public.[3] (See chapter 10.)

My goals in writing this book are to discuss some of the reasons for this shift in patients' perceptions, as well as to describe the principles you need to understand before making a decision regarding your health. The final decisions as to how to prevent disease, whether to be screened for an illness, take a diagnostic test or a treatment recommended by a medical or alternative health practitioner are yours.

In order for you to make the right decisions, that is, decisions which lead to more good than harm, you must be armed with the knowledge required to discard hype, marketing, and peer pressure and to evaluate the scientific evidence behind the recommendation. Although this might sound intimidating, the principles behind good scientific evidence are fairly simple. All you need is an open mind and knowledge of the steps required to evaluate evidence.

Health care consumers who have this approach will not swallow pills that have not, in good studies, been shown to do more good than harm. They will insist on real evidence that a serious condition like autism is caused by immunization before they stop their children from being vaccinated. They will look at the overall benefits of cholesterol-lowering medications, as well as the risks. Before taking their seriously depressed teenagers off the antidepressants that have been helping them lead normal lives, parents will insist on good evidence which refutes the benefits of the medication.

In other words, asking the right questions and understanding how to evaluate the evidence behind the answers will help you to make the right decisions in caring for your health. In addition, fewer unnecessary tests, medications, surgical procedures, and hospitalizations will save patients and taxpayers considerable amounts of money.

References:

[1.] McKeown, T. *The Role of Medicine: Dream, Mirage, or Nemesis?* The Nuffield Provincial Hospitals Trust, 1976, p31

[2.] Illich, I., *Medical Nemesis*, McClelland and Stewart, 1975, p11

[3.] Verghese, A. *New York Times*, 12/8/02, from Medscape Primary Care.

CHAPTER 2

Why Have So Many Patients Turned to Alternative Health Care Providers?

In all probability there is no single answer to the question of why patients have turned to alternative health care providers. However, several identifiable factors influence the increase in the use of unproven treatments and practices. These factors include the roles of media, education, doctors and pharmaceutical companies, and government.

Perhaps the best example of the effect the media have on the public's health care decision-making is shown in the following case, in which the media erroneously supported a physician's unusual treatment.

At the end of 1997, an Italian cancer physician achieved prominence when he claimed to have cured thousands of cancer patients with a mixture of medications and vitamins. He said that this therapy had few side effects. The treatment had never been studied in either animals or humans, and no reports concerning it had been published in medical journals.

Because the treatment was expensive (about five thousand dollars U.S. per patient per month) the Italian government was asked to pay for it. In view of the lack of evidence of its effectiveness, the government refused.

The doctor's patients challenged the government decision. The media made this front-page news. All the characteristics of a great story were at hand: a potentially life-threatening disease; an old, trusted cancer doctor who had become a hero trying to care for his sick patients; a fight against a government only interested in saving money; and a medical profession which puts more emphasis on the need for better evidence than on helping sick patients. There were about three hundred newspaper articles and more than fifty television interviews about the story. Because of the media coverage, many cancer patients chose the new treatment.

The health authorities were very surprised when the courts ruled that this treatment should be covered by the government health plan. The media portrayed the judge as a brave hero, fighting the government and the medical profession. Many of the media's articles were negative about the medical profession's opposition to the new "cure"; those doctors who tried to promote research on the treatment were labelled as patients' enemies.

The government, while paying for the treatment, was able to insist on evidence based on solid research—the results of which showed that not only did the treatment have no beneficial effect on the cancers, it also had side effects.[1]

Paying for the treatments and the research cost the Italian taxpayers twenty million dollars. In addition, it is possible that some patients may have died—having given up effective cancer therapy because the media publicized this unproven therapy. Other patients may have opted for *no* therapy after this "cure" was shown to be useless.

Shortly after this media frenzy, a study interviewing Italian cancer patients was undertaken. When choosing a treatment, the patients felt that the advice of a trusted doctor was more important than scientific evidence, and two-thirds said they would try unproven treatments. Most of these cancer patients said they got their information about various treatments from television and radio, and about one-quarter of respondents got their information from newspapers. Half said they had not discussed the new cancer therapy with their specialist; those who had said they were less likely to try an unproven therapy.[2]

An editorial comment in the journal in which this story was described concluded:

"This sad story has revealed how poorly the mass media (with a few notable exceptions) understand medical matters. It also showed, not surprisingly in a country that is neglecting science in schools, a profound lack of knowledge among the public of how advances in medicine are achieved."[3]

In a British study that examined what medical news is newsworthy, the researchers determined which articles published in major medical journals the media had selected.[4]

Results showed that newspapers under-reported studies involving randomized controlled trials (RCTs)—in other words, studies considered to be the best evidence—and were likelier to report dramatic case reports or observational, uncontrolled research, which are much more prone to bias. Another study showed that bad news was much more likely than good news to be published in the newspapers, even though the press releases from medical journals contained an equal number of good news and bad news studies.[5]

The researchers who reviewed the media reports concluded: "We are concerned that many aspects of medical research are not represented in newspapers." The article stressed that newspapers have an important effect on policy-makers, consumers of health services, and the population in general.

Under-reporting the best scientific evidence and over-reporting bad news will have to change if media coverage is to have a beneficial effect.

The problem caused by a lack of accurate, evidence-based media reporting of health issues is not restricted to Europe. Recently, a major U.S. weekly magazine had a special section on "How your mind can heal your body." Although much of the reporting was reasonable, the magazine gave one and a half pages to a physician they called "a guru of alternative medicine."[6] In his article he described breathing exercises and meditation as solutions for depression. In addition, he claimed that certain nutritional deficiencies "may be a factor in childhood autism, attention deficit hyperactivity disorder, bipolar disorder, and depression." Although he did write that there should be research in these areas, he acknowledged that he is already recommending certain fatty acid supplements for the treatment of some of these diseases.

The problem with this material appearing in a major U.S. magazine is that people with the diseases he mentioned, most of which have treatments already shown by RCTs to be effective, might not seek appropriate care and may try unproven and possibly dangerous treatments.

As Theodore R. Marmor, professor of public policy at the Yale School of Management, has written: "Most mainstream North American journalists regard apparently dramatic stories as more their subject than complicated explanations of complicated programs. Pressure groups provide stories and claims that serve their interests and should be regarded with caution."[7]

The news is not all bad, however. There are attempts by some in the media to promote better reporting about health issues.

In a recent column in the *Toronto Star*, ombudsman Don Sellar wrote: "This corner has long contended that *The Star* and other media outlets need to be more rigorous in the reporting of research studies.... For example, was the work independent and free of commercial taint? Did a ketchup-maker fund the study 'proving' tomatoes have properties that might forestall cancer? Was it good science? Were enough people studied?.... Please, when reporting on science—especially when debate is so hot—let's give readers more information, not less."[8]

Similarly, a recent editorial in the *New York Times*, describing research showing a newborn screening test for cancer to be useless (even though it had been used on millions of babies), discussed the value of other screening tests. "A key issue is whether the tests are finding a lot of tumours that would never become dangerous but cannot be distinguished from tumours that could become deadly, thereby causing many patients to undergo the risks of surgery, radiation or chemotherapy for no good reason.... Many tests have been adopted mostly on faith."[9]

While such an editorial is encouraging, it is clear that the media still has a long way to go. A recent article in a major U.S. medical journal reviewed news coverage about screening mammography for low-risk women in their forties for the primary prevention of breast cancer. The authors found differences in how the news media reported on these issues. The stories about breast cancer screening were "remarkable for the extent to which politicians and advocacy groups were represented."[10]

Fewer than half the stories reported some of the side effects of screening low-risk women in their forties, such as over-diagnosis, the resultant unnecessary biopsies, and anxiety.

As Don Sellar wrote, "media outlets need to be more rigorous in the reporting of research studies." For this to happen, more medical reporters and editors need to be better informed about what constitutes good evidence, and they need to ask the tough questions.

In describing the enormous impact of the media on the public's health care decisions, one realizes that the media have to be placed in context with our culture. Medical sociologists have been studying these issues for many years.

In her book *Essays in Medical Sociology*, the eminent medical sociologist Dr. Renée Fox points out that in all societies, health, illness, and medicine are very important. She writes that science, magic, and religion are all involved in how people think about these issues, and that, universally, medical practitioners have considerable influence and prestige because of what she calls the "magico-religious system."[11] In many cultures, what determines the health, illness, symptoms, and "cure" of a patient is the belief the patient has in the healer. For many, this "belief" amounts to faith, or religious belief, that the practitioner has magical skills.

Dr. Fox also discusses the "competence gap," described by Dr. Talcott Parsons, a leading medical sociologist. The competence gap that exists between physician and patient exists because one is a trained expert in matters of health and illness and the other is not; as Parsons writes, "the physician and the patient form a collectivity based on their joint commitment to the recovery of the sick person." In order for this to be achieved, Dr. Parsons points out that mutual trust between the doctor and patient is necessary.[12]

Medical sociologists write about "science, magic, and religion" as the major ways in which health care issues are addressed in a society. They confirm that doctors and patients are bound to each other by the competency gap and by their joint commitment to the recovery of the patient.

There will always be a competency gap between doctors and patients, although it is likely that cultural change can shrink the gap; but such change can only come about if "magic" and "religion" become less important as the major media and science (or evidence) take a more prominent role. Culture is defined as "the arts, customs, and institutions of a nation, people, or group." The origin is from the Latin for "growing." Cultural attitudes change and are not static. The roles of women and minority groups have changed dramatically in the last century. A major force toward cultural change is the educational system, which in most of the developed world does not use problem-solving, answer-seeking approaches to teaching children, but instead concentrates on didactic authoritarian approaches, not only in what it teaches but also in how it teaches. In fact, it is unlikely that studying to be a teacher in college or university prepares teachers for an evidence-based approach. Education is defined as "the process of teaching or learning, the theory and practice of teaching, or training in a particular subject." The origin of the word is from the Latin *educare*, or "lead out." Good teachers lead their students out of ignorance; the best teachers teach their students how to learn.

In the course of writing two previous books on evidence-based approaches to helping children with learning difficulties, it became abundantly clear to me that teacher training colleges do not teach teachers how to evaluate evidence, especially regarding how to help children with reading problems or attention deficit hyperactivity disorder. For one thing, very little research in educational remediation is based on properly conducted RCTs (see Chapter 4). For another, teachers are not systematically taught how to evaluate the quality of the evidence that one mode of teaching is better than another. This explains why, decades ago, teaching reading by phonics was replaced by the whole word recognition system. There was no evidence that the new system was better, and yet educators everywhere adopted it because it seemed like a good idea. Because reading skills in primary and high school students are now significantly lower after decades of using the whole word recognition system, many school boards are mandating a move back to the use of phonics.

In fact, for students with proven reading problems there are now excellent randomized controlled trials showing that phonics is the best way to remediate the problem.

The "open concept" classroom was another educational concept which was widely followed without good evidence showing its value.

Having reviewed how the media and the educational system sustain the uncritical approach people adopt when making decisions about their health care, it is important to review other factors which support this lack of insistence on sound evidence.

An important component of this deficit is the pharmaceutical industry. More than forty per cent of people in the United States take at least one prescription medication, and almost one in five take at least three medications.[13] In one Canadian province, over one year, two-thirds of the population received at least one prescription; the mean number of prescriptions per patient that year was 8.2.[14] Many of these drugs are not only well worth the money patients spend on them, but have also been shown in good scientific studies to be relatively safe and to prevent, cure, or alleviate the symptoms of acute or chronic diseases. This is not always the case, however. As the recent evidence shows, some of the newer anti-inflammatory prescription drugs are not only dangerous but also much more expensive—and no more effective—than over-the-counter arthritis medications.

Patients were willing to spend the extra money for these drugs for two reasons. The first reason was the intense, dramatic advertisements showing that these pills could restore a normal life to the patient suffering from the pain and limitations of arthritis. The second reason was that their doctors prescribed the medication. Television commercials showed attractive actors swimming, playing golf and tennis, smiling. Patients who saw these advertisements would often pressure their physicians to write the prescription, and most often the physicians did.

Why do drug companies spend so many millions of dollars on these advertisements? Because they are effective at selling the product. The pharmaceutical industry is among the most profitable in the world. Although much of the money earned is spent on research and the development of new medications, very high profits going to shareholders are realized even *after* the money is spent on research.

Why do so many doctors prescribe some medications before they have been shown, over time, to do more good than harm? There are several reasons. The first is that even though most physicians keep themselves up-to-date and try to practice evidence-based medicine, some of the articles they read in medical journals are biased in favour of the product studied. This is because much of the funding for medical research comes from the pharmaceutical and surgical equipment industries. A recent study showed that published industry-funded research is much more likely to be associated with pro-industry results.[15] This is not only because the medical or surgical product was necessarily more effective and safe, although most are. There are several reasons why negative results are not published as readily. First, as more than half of biomedical company executives recently admitted, their research agreements with universities included restrictions on communicating negative results. Second, new products may need to be on the market for some time before serious side effects are discovered. The follow-up and reporting of these potentially harmful aspects of products has been poor, and physicians, companies, and governments have been lax in this regard, as the Vioxx story has revealed. Third, even when drug companies are aware that a potentially major profit-maker might be harmful, the profit motive can delay action as long as possible; profits could be in the billions of dollars. Of course, delaying bad information has led to class action lawsuits, which can then cost the company significant amounts of money.

One must also question the relationship between the drug companies and the prescribing physicians. Doctors have contact with the pharmaceutical companies early in their careers. In 2002, the industry spent approximately one-third of its revenues on "selling and administration."[16] In 2001, there were nearly ninety thousand drug detailers—those who meet individually with physicians to promote their products—in the United States. Drug companies give physicians gifts such as pens and pads with the product or company's name, as well as paying large honoraria to prominent doctors who promote their products. They support travel and other expenses for doctors to attend medical conferences. Most practising physicians receive free samples; the patient who receives the sample is more likely to ask for the sample to be prescribed even though there may be less expensive, equally safe and effective medications available.

Drug companies also support the medical conferences which doctors attend for their continuing education. Some of the authors of clinical guidelines for practising doctors have had financial ties with the companies whose drugs the guideline may recommend.

Most physicians feel they can resist the incentives to promote a particular product, even if they accept free pens or trips to conferences. One study reviewed the statistics to see whether this is true. In fact, doctors were *likelier* to use the promoted product, even though there may have been equally safe, effective, and less expensive alternatives.[17]

In general, industry support for medical research has been invaluable, leading to many new treatments which have helped numerous patients.

However, because the connections between companies, medical school researchers, doctors' organizations, individual physicians, and governments can have actual and potentially negative results as well as positive, doctors' organizations, governments, and companies are attempting to strengthen standards. In an excellent article entitled "Doctors and Drug Companies," Doctor David Blumenthal, a professor at the Institute for Health Policy at Harvard Medical School, states: "Taken together, this series of private and public pronouncements seems to embrace the view that relationships between some drug companies and physicians are ethically appropriate, often beneficial, and certainly unavoidable and that the challenge for the medical profession, drug companies, and the government is to contain those relationships within acceptable boundaries and to avoid certain egregious and possibly illegal practices."[18]

According to Doctor Blumenthal, critics claim it is essentially up to the medical profession and individual doctors not to accept anything of financial value, no matter how trivial, from drug companies.

What is the role of governments in ensuring that drug products available to patients are effective, relatively safe, and affordable? The answer to this question is complicated by the close relationship between governments and the drug industry, especially in the United States. The pharmaceutical industry has the largest lobby in Washington and gives sizable amounts of money to political campaigns.[19] This is believed to have a major impact on government decision-making regarding pharmaceuticals. For example, the U.S. Food and Drug Administration (FDA) does not insist that drug companies test their new products against old products created for the same disease, even when some of these products are already on the market. Thus, with effective advertising, new products may outsell well-recognized, safe, effective, and less expensive drugs. In fact, the older product might turn out to be safer than the new one.

The FDA is but one of many scientific and technical advisory government committees in the United States.

Recently, the Union of Concerned Scientists reported that "there is strong documentation of a wide-ranging effort to manipulate the government's scientific advisory system to prevent the appearance of advice that might run counter to the administration's political agenda."[20]

Merrill Goozner, director of the Integrity in Science project at the Centre for Science in the Public Interest, described the problems and a potential solution: "People confront dizzying choices in health care everyday: are brand-name drugs better than generic versions?... How serious are the side effects of a drug and how do its benefits compare to, say, losing 30 pounds?... To make rational choices, doctors and consumers need the FDA and other agencies to be independent arbiters of not just the safety and efficacy of new drugs and devices, but of their relative medical usefulness and economic viability. Moreover, the medical oversight system needs a new ethic—one that scrupulously adheres to a standard that says its studies and decisions have been made entirely free of commercial bias and conflicts of interest. Sadly, that is very far from the situation today. Drug and device companies sponsor most clinical trials; FDA advisory panels are loaded with scientists tied to private companies; corporate user fees help finance the FDA, that is conducting reviews; doctors get most of their medical information either from sales representatives of drug companies or corporate-sponsored continuing medical education; and the companies are given primary responsibility for post-marketing safety surveillance of their own products."[21]

To solve these problems, Goozner recommends an independent arm of the FDA. This group would ensure that after a company applies to market a drug based on preliminary safety and efficacy studies, a protocol would be established that compares the new drug to a placebo as well as to other treatments; in addition, post-marketing studies following longer-term safety testing would be financed independently of the drug's manufacturer. Goozner also recommends some restrictions on direct advertising to consumers. "Not until the system of medical approval and information is returned to objective hands will doctors and consumers be able to make the wisest and most cost-effective medical choices."

The relationship between drug companies and the federal government is somewhat different in Canada. The data used to approve new pharmaceutical products is considered confidential under the Canadian Access to Information Act. The Therapeutic Products Directorate (TPD) will only release this information with the manufacturer's consent, whereas the FDA will release results from unpublished pre-clinical and clinical trials if requested. Although there is a concerted effort in Canada to release more information about clinical trials, a recent study suggests that these new attempts are insufficient.[22]

One difference between the U.S. and Canadian governments and the drug industry has to do with the price of drugs. Drug prices in Canada are substantially lower than those in the U.S. That is because the U.S. is the only country in the developed world which does not regulate drug prices. In addition, direct-to-consumer advertising of prescription medications, legal in the U.S., is illegal in Canada, although companies seem to be testing the limits of the law in Canada. Cable and satellite TV, as well as print media and the Internet, have had, in all likelihood, a huge impact on the consumer in Canada as well as the U.S.

Another difference is the length of time it takes to approve a drug in the U.S. compared to Canada. New drugs are approved more quickly in the U.S. than in Canada. Pressure to speed up the Canadian process is coming from two main sources. Patient groups that hear about new treatments approved in the U.S. which are not yet available in Canada put pressure on the Canadian government. Even more pressure is applied by pharmaceutical company lobbyists who are concerned about profits. Concern has been expressed that putting more money into speeding up the approval process might be at the expense of the post-marketing surveillance system. "To satisfy all of its various stakeholders Health Canada will have to balance timeliness and safety. How it goes about this delicate task will be interesting to watch."[23] Post-marketing surveillance in Canada will become more transparent, since in mid-2005 Health Canada announced that adverse drug reactions will be made public on its website.

Finally, the editors of medical journals have begun to realize that they must be more rigorous in ensuring that what they publish is scientifically accurate and not susceptible to bias. If the authors of medical journal articles have a conflict of interest—if they have received personal gain from the company whose product is described in the article—it is possible that the benefits may be stressed and the risks suppressed. The International Committee of Medical Journal Editors has issued the following statement: "Conflict of interest exists when an author (or the author's institution), reviewer, or editor has financial or personal relationships that inappropriately influence (bias) his or her actions...."[24]

Because this statement is felt to be too general, individual journals are developing more rigorous policies. For example, the *Canadian Medical Association Journal*'s new policy states the following: "Commentaries and narrative reviews or other similar articles, whether commissioned or spontaneously submitted, will not be accepted for consideration for publication if any author has any financial investments (such as equity, shares, derivatives, bonds, but excluding publicly traded mutual funds), receives royalties or similar payments, that in total over the past year has exceeded US $10,000 per company; or holds a patent (or is likely to or has applied for one or more) in a company that markets a product (or a competitor's product) mentioned in the article. Nor will we accept for publication papers by authors who are employed by such companies, who have a contractual relationship of any type with such companies, or who are named officers or board members of such companies."

In summary, if the media, medical school researchers, doctors' organizations, individual physicians, medical journals, and government drug agencies all insist on rigorous, objective scientific data perhaps there will be fewer Vioxx scenarios. It is hoped that drug companies will also apply more ethical marketing practices before they are forced to do so when class action legal settlements cut into their profits.

Finally, when the public is armed with the information to make the right decisions in caring for health, people will take those actions for which there is good evidence that the benefits outweigh the risks.

References:

1. Remuzzi, G., Schieppati, A., "Lessons from the Di Bella affair—Commentary." *The Lancet,* 353: 1289–1290, 1999

2. Passalacqua, R., Campione, F., Caminiti, C., et al. "Patients' opinions, feelings, and attitudes after a campaign to promote Di Bella therapy." *The Lancet,* 353: 1310–14, 1999

3. Remuzzi, G., Schieppati, A., "Lessons from the Di Bella Affair—Commentary."

4. White, P.D. "Bad press for doctors: 21 year survey of three national newspapers." *British Medical Journal* (BMJ), 323, 782–3, 2002

55. Egger, M. "What is newsworthy? Longtitudinal study of the reporting of medical research in two British newspapers." *BMJ,* 325, 81–84, 2000

6. Weil, A. "Mother nature's little helpers." *Time*, Jan.20, 2003, p42–43.

7. Marmor, T. "Medicare: Suspect messages." *The Globe and Mail*, Feb.12/02

8. Sellar, D. "Let's give medical stories a checkup." *Toronto Star*, Oct.5/02

9. Editorial, *New York Times*, April 19/02

10. Schwartz, L.M., and Woloshin, S. "News Media Coverage of Screening Mammography for Women in their 40's and Tamoxifen for Primary Prevention of Breast Cancer." *Journal of American Medical Association* (JAMA), 287, 3136–3142, 2002

11. Fox, R.C. *Essays in Medical Sociology: Journeys into the Field.* John Wiley and Sons, 1979, p472

12. Ibid, p500

13. National Center for Health Statistics Report, quoted in the *New York Times*, Dec.3, 2004

14. Quinn, K., Baker, M.J., Evans, B., "A population-wide profile of prescription drug use in Saskatchewan, 1989." *Canadian Medical Association Journal* (CMAJ), 146(12), 2177–2186, 1992

15. Bhandari, M., Busse, J.W., Jackowski, D., et.al. "Association Between Industry Funding and Statistically Significant Pro-Industry Findings in Medical and Surgical Randomized Trials." *CMAJ* 170(4), 477–80, 2004

16. Reinhardt, U.E. "An information infrastructure for the pharmaceutical market." *Health Affairs* (Millwood), 23(1), 107–12, 2004

17. Wazana, A. "Physicians and the pharmaceutical industry: is a gift ever just a gift?" *JAMA* 283, 373–80, 2000.

18. Blumenthal, D. "Doctors and Drug Companies." *New England Journal of Medicine*, 351:18, 1885–1890, 2004

19. Aaron C., Lincoln, T. "The other drug war 2003: Drug companies deploy an army of 675 lobbyists to protect profits." Washington, D.C.: *The Public Citizen Congress Watch*; June 2003

20. Steinbrook, R. "Science, Politics, and Federal Advisory Committees." *New England Journal of Medicine.* 350; 14, 1454–1460, 2004

21. OpEd Contributor: "Overdozed and Oversold." *New York Times*, Dec.21/2004

22. Lexchin, J., Mintzes, B. "Transparency in drug regulation: Mirage or oasis?" *CMAJ*, 171(11), 1363–1365, 2004

23. Lexchin, J. "New directions in drug approval." *CMAJ*, 171(3), 229–230, 2004

24. Editorial, "Conflicts of interests and investments." *CMAJ*, 171(11), 1313, 2004

CHAPTER 3

Preventing Illness:
How to Make the Right Decisions

We are all bombarded with information about how to stay healthy: lose weight, stop smoking, exercise, have regular checkups, etc. Most often the advice is sound, based on reasonably good evidence. Because this is not always the case, it is important that the public be shown how to evaluate whether a preventive manoeuvre is worthwhile.

Some patients are afraid to ask questions of their doctors; some doctors (hopefully a minority) feel that when a patient asks questions the doctors' authority is challenged. While it is true that not all physicians have the sensitivity and interpersonal skills required to be part of the patients' evidence-gathering process, change is at hand. For some time now, most medical schools and post-graduate programs have been stressing the importance of good communication skills and have devoted educational time to enhancing the doctors' ability to appreciate the patients' need to know. Most doctors currently in practice are aware that their patients are often better informed than those of previous decades, largely due to much wider use of the Internet. As a result, doctors are usually not surprised when asked about a diagnosis, a test, or a treatment.

If you approach your family doctor or specialist in a non-confrontational manner, e.g. "I saw on the Internet that there is controversy about the PSA test," most physicians will not be offended if you express your wish not to have the test done at this time. Those who are offended are probably not your best choice of doctor. On the other hand, if your doctor takes the time to explain why, in your particular case, given your symptoms and what was found on physical examination the test might be reasonable, although the choice is still yours, that physician might be your best choice.

The best combination is a patient who asks questions in a non-challenging manner and a physician who is proud to be part of the evidence-seeking process.

This chapter deals with prevention: staying healthy and preventing disease.

Prevention

Your neighbour Margaret's three-and-a-half-year-old son has recently been diagnosed with autism. You suspected something was wrong because he seemed behind in his development. He did not speak and didn't seem to understand when people spoke to him. He didn't make eye contact, flapped his hands in an odd way, and always seemed to want to watch the Shopping Channel on TV. Margaret is sure the problem was caused by the measles, mumps and rubella (MMR) vaccination he received when he was younger. She got this information from the Internet.

Challenge
The problem you are facing is that your daughter's doctor wants her to have her MMR vaccination at her next visit. What should you do? Preventing measles, mumps and rubella, or German measles, is important, because these diseases can produce serious complications, even death. At the same time, in Margaret's son you have seen how autism has affected the whole family.

Margaret got her information from the Internet. You type in the keywords "autism and vaccination" and you find a number of websites. Many of them, government-run or from medical journals, state that there is no relation between MMR and autism. On the other hand, you notice others that say there is a connection. The questions you need answered are:

1) Is MMR effective at preventing disease?
2) Does MMR cause autism?

This challenge is not meant to dwell in detail on the possible link but is merely to be used as an example of what evidence is required before taking a step to prevent disease.

The first step to take in deciding if a measure to maintain health and prevent disease will do more good than harm is to ask whether valid randomized controlled trials (RCTs) have been done. An RCT is a study designed to answer the following question: will a group of people given the intervention do better than a group who is given a placebo or no intervention? Randomization (the process whereby individuals are randomly allocated to receive or not receive an experimental preventive, therapeutic, or diagnostic procedure) is important to ensure that the two groups will be as similar as possible. Similarity between groups is essential in order to prevent an erroneous interpretation of results which might arise not because of the preventive manoeuvre but because the groups were different to start with. For example, if children given MMR vaccinations come from richer homes than children who don't receive the vaccine, increased cases of measles, mumps, and rubella in the unvaccinated children might have more to do with overcrowding and poor nutrition than with not receiving the vaccine. In addition to being comparable with regard to social class, the groups should also be comparable in age. If by chance the vaccinated group is much younger, they might still get measles, mumps, or rubella—because the vaccine is only effective in children old enough to build up antibodies to the vaccine and therefore to the diseases.

The best way to be certain that the vaccinated and unvaccinated groups are similar at the beginning of the study is to do a randomized controlled trial. Once informed consent has been given, every patient has to have an equal opportunity to receive either the vaccine or a placebo (an inactive substance that has no treatment value). In order for this to happen the allocation to one group or the other has to be strictly by chance, like a coin toss: if you toss the coin often enough, you come up with heads half the time and with tails half the time.

It is also very important that the randomization not be biased: for example, in one study comparing anti-fever medication with sponging, the nurses knew which patient was to be assigned to which group by looking at the chart number. It is possible that, in their desire to be helpful, they might have assigned the sicker patients to the medication if they felt the medication was more effective. At the end of the study, if one treatment was found to be equivalent to the other, the results could have been biased. If patients at the outset in *both* groups had been equally ill, one treatment might actually have been more effective than the other. Thus in the process of randomization, in order for the groups to be the same at the beginning, it is important that the researchers be "blinded"—they should not know in advance to which group the patient is being assigned.

Sometimes a new treatment is so striking in its early research that a randomized controlled trial cannot be done. For example, when penicillin was discovered it was very apparent that many patients who previously would have died from serious bacterial infections were not only alive after penicillin treatment, but were completely back to normal. In this case the evidence consists of comparing data from the period before the intervention with data from patients who received the treatment.

The reason it is important to have information from RCTs and/or dramatic differences between times with and without MMR is for people like Margaret's neighbour to know whether the vaccine is effective. In other words, do children who get MMR have fewer cases of measles, mumps, and rubella than children who do not? Are there fewer deaths and serious complications like brain damage from measles, sterility in males from mumps, and fewer babies born with congenital rubella syndrome to those individuals who have been vaccinated?

In the case of MMR, the answers are clear: measles, mumps, and rubella and their complications have virtually disappeared from the developed world since MMR's almost universal use in preschoolers. For example, in the U.S., between three and four million cases of measles were reported each year before the widespread use of vaccine. In that era, there were several thousand deaths from the complications of measles each year. By 1982, about twenty years after the initiation of measles immunization, there were fewer than 1500 cases, and by 2001 there were fewer than two hundred. In 2000 ninety-nine per cent of all counties in the U.S. reported no cases of measles.[1]

In addition to the dramatic evidence described above, there have also been RCTs demonstrating the effectiveness of MMR.[2]

You have been given the information that the vaccine is effective. However, because of your concern that the vaccine might cause autism in your daughter, you may still be reluctant to have your daughter immunized. How does one answer the question as to whether MMR causes autism?

Good evidence that a disease is or is not caused by a suspected agent (causation) can be obtained by a cohort study, in which one follows a large group of patients exposed to the presumed agent (MMR), and determines whether this group has a significantly higher incidence of the disease (autism) than a group which does not receive the agent. In one study, more than half a million children (eighty-two per cent received MMR) were followed for some years; there was no increase in autism in those who were vaccinated.[3]

Another approach in determining causation is the case-control study. In this type of research the investigators assess patients with the disease (cases) and compare them to individuals without the disease (controls) matched as closely as possibly for factors which might influence whether they get the disease, like age, gender, social class, etc. With regard to assessing the potential effect of MMR as a cause of autism, a number of investigators have studied cases and controls. If MMR were a potential cause, there should be a significantly greater number of autistic children who received MMR (cases) than non-autistic children (controls). In one case-control study, 1294 patients with autism and 4469 controls, matched on age, gender, and physician's practice were studied. Of the cases of autism, seventy-eight per cent had received MMR. Of the non-autistic controls, eighty-two per cent had received MMR. Thus, fewer autistic children had received MMR when compared with non-autistic controls.[4] A number of other researchers have found the same results—in fact, there are no cohort or case-control studies showing that more autistic patients received MMR than non-autistic persons. This is good evidence that MMR does not cause autism.

When it comes to assessing evidence of causation, the least convincing type of investigation is the case series. In this kind of research, an investigator studies a group of patients and comes up with a hypothesis as to what caused their condition. This is the type of study that suggested a link between MMR and autism. In 1998 an article was published in *The Lancet*, a famous British medical journal, which described twelve children with autism who also had problems with their gastrointestinal systems. The authors hypothesized that MMR caused bowel inflammation, which then led to autism.[5] The media's quick announcement of this dramatic news led to the immunization rate in the U.K. dropping from over ninety-two per cent to less than eighty per cent.[6] In turn, this drop in immunization resulted in a dramatic increase in measles as well as some measles-related deaths. Immunization rates also fell somewhat in other parts of the developed world.

The problem with this paper linking MMR to autism goes even deeper. Researchers can make mistakes. In this case, however, there was a major conflict of interest on the part of the principal investigator: it appears as though he had received a significant amount of money to "find" evidence of a link between MMR and autism. This money was given to him by a group of parents who believed there was a link and who had taken legal action against the manufacturer of MMR.[7] Once this fact was made public, other investigators involved with this report sent a letter to the editor of *The Lancet* disclaiming their support of the so-called relationship between MMR and autism.

So, if cohort and case-control studies, considered better evidence of causation than case series, find no relationship between MMR and autism, and the one report of a possible relationship is flawed both scientifically and by conflict of interest, how else can one explain what appears to be a dramatic increase in autism?

The prevalence of diagnosed autism has risen. In one study autism was diagnosed in three per ten thousand children in 1991–92 and in fifty-two per ten thousand in 2001–2002.[8] The authors make the important point that this may not be a true increase but rather that autism was under-diagnosed in the past. The authors of another study, which found an eightfold increase from 1976 to 1997, state that the increase occurred "after the introduction of broader, more precise diagnostic criteria, increased availability of services, and increased awareness of autism."[9] It would appear that the main reason for the so-called increase in autism is that the condition clinicians used to diagnose as "mental retardation" is now being given the appropriate diagnosis. A study showing that "mental retardation" has decreased in prevalence by about the same number as "autism" has increased is evidence that proves this theory.[10]

Another factor causing parents to be concerned about the link between MMR and autism is that the most striking abnormalities of that condition appear to show themselves shortly after the vaccination. This temporal link makes the connection seem plausible. However, the relationship is much more apparent than real, because it is only after the first year of life (around the time of the first MMR dose) that parents' expectations for rapid development become high—walking, talking, and more socialization are all expected to be present after this period. However, many of the features of autism were probably present but not considered worrisome before this time: absence of eye contact, no social smile, no response to being hugged.

In summary, perhaps the most important development in preventing illness (in addition to public health
measures such as purification of drinking water and reg-
ulating food quality and sanitation) has been the
widespread implementation of immunization programs.
In making the decision to adopt a preventive measure,
knowledgeable consumers will ask if there is evidence
from randomized controlled trials that the benefits outweigh the risks. As there may not be RCTs for some
preventive measures, there should be cohort studies or
case-control studies showing that individuals who have
the preventive intervention are better off than those who
don't. Unless there are dramatic differences in the incidence of a disorder before and after an intervention is
adopted, or between communities which do or do not
use the preventive measure, it is better to wait. It is also
best to wait until case series suggesting that something
works (or is dangerous) have been proven valid by RCTs,
cohort, or case-control studies.

References:

[1.] Meissner, H.C., Strebel, P.M., and Orenstein, W.A. "Measles
Vaccines and the Potential for Worldwide Eradication of
Measles." *Pediatrics*, 114:4, 1065–1069, 2004

[2.] Gold, R., Martell, A. *Childhood Immunizations in The Canadian
Guide to Clinical Preventive Health Care*. Health Canada,
1994: 372–384

[3.] Madsen K.M., Hviid, A., Vestergaard, M., et al. "MMR vaccination and autism—a population-based follow-up study."
Ugesker Laeger, 164(49), 5741–4, 2002

4. Smeeth, L., Cook, C., Fombonne, E., et al. "MMR vaccination and pervasive developmental disorders: a case-control study." *The Lancet*, 364(9438), 963–9, 2004

5. Wakefield, A.J., Murch, S.H., Anthony, A., et al. "Ileal-lymphoid-nodular hyperplasia, non-specific colitis, and pervasive developmental disorder in children." *The Lancet*, 351, 637–41, 1998

6. Embree, J. "Ethics in research: Immunization and autism links." *Paediatric Child Health,* 9(6), 373–374, 2004

7. Ibid.

8. Gurney, J.G., Fritz, M.S., Ness, K.K., et al. "Analysis of prevalence trends of autism spectrum disorder in Minnesota." *Archives of Pediatrics & Adolescent Medicine*, 157(7), 622–7, 2003

9. Barbaresi, W.J., Katusic, S.K., Colligan, R.C., et al. "The incidence of autism in Olmsted County, Minnesota, 1976–1997: results from a population-based study." *Archives of Pediatrics & Adolescent Medicine*, 159(1), 37–44, 2005

10. Fombonne, E. "The prevalence of autism." *JAMA*, 289,(1), 87–89, 2003

CHAPTER 4

Staying Healthy:
What about Screening Tests?

"Screening" is an attempt to find disorders or risk factors for diseases among apparently healthy persons in the community. The term "screening" usually refers to groups of people, like office workers who are offered free blood-pressure checks by the company's nurse. The phrase most often used to define a screening test done one-to-one in the doctor's office—when the patient comes in for a routine checkup or for a totally unrelated problem—is "case-finding." An example of case-finding is when a patient comes in to be treated for a bladder infection, the physician notices that the patient has never had a cholesterol test and orders it even though the patient has no history of heart disease.

Challenge
You are a healthy fifty-year-old male and your doctor recommends that you have a prostate-specific antigen (PSA) screening test. In addition, you have seen on an early-morning TV program how a well-known politician's life

was saved by having his prostate cancer treated early,
thanks to his PSA *test. What information do you need in*
order to decide whether to have the test?

Ideally, the benefits vs. harm of a screening test should
have been studied in a randomized controlled trial.
Healthy men, aged fifty years or more, should be randomly allocated to either have or not have the PSA test.
Both groups should then be followed for a long enough
period to determine whether the screened group lived a
longer, better life because of early treatment of prostate
cancer than did the unscreened group.

There have not been many RCTs of screening programs; when they have been done, the results are often
disappointing. For example, breast self-examination
(BSE) was widely promoted for many years so that
women could identify breast cancer early enough to save
their lives. It was only after two randomized trials
involving close to four hundred thousand women
showed no significant difference in breast cancer mortality between the women who did regular BSE and those
who did not that BSE was no longer widely promoted. In
those studies almost twice as many biopsies which
turned out to be normal were done in the screened
group compared to the controls.[1] In addition to the pain
and cost associated with the large number of biopsies in
the screened group, one can imagine the anxiety when a
woman finds a lump and thus suspects she has cancer. If
there was a real improvement in the duration and quality of life in the screened group, then the pain, cost, and
anxiety associated with the false positive tests would no

doubt be considered worthwhile. It was not until these results were published that it became clear that BSE was associated with more harm than good.

In addition to whether or not RCTs of the screening test have been done, it is important to know whether early diagnosis really makes a difference. In other words, if our fifty-year-old male with no symptoms of prostate problems does in fact have a prostate cancer, does diagnosing and treating it before symptoms develop make a difference in the duration and quality of his life?

One of the problems in deciding whether early diagnosis of prostate cancer makes a difference is that the disease is so common.[2] About twenty per cent of men whose average age is fifty, and who die of other causes, are found to have prostate cancer at autopsy; when men get to their eighties, the number jumps to forty-three per cent. In other words, the disease is so common that the comment "more men die with prostate cancer than from prostate cancer" is frequently expressed.

In one study, a group of men aged fifty to sixty-nine who had both PSA screening and rectal exam were studied; another group served as controls, which means they had neither the PSA nor the rectal exam. The groups were followed for a number of years. Although there were more cancers identified in the screened group, there were no differences in total survival or in survival with prostate cancer between the groups.[3] In other words, the unscreened group lived as long as the screened group.

Although this study suggests early diagnosis does not make a difference in mortality, there were some problems with the study design. For example, although it was stated to be a RCT, the researchers knew in advance which person was to be screened. The design of the study specified that every sixth man aged fifty to sixty-nine in the doctors' general practices was to be screened. Thus it is possible that some patients with a family history of prostate cancer might have been excluded from the study because the researchers wanted them screened. This potential bias in the study design makes the results showing no benefit to screening less certain.

If there is no good evidence that current treatment for the problem helps, what about potential harm to those who are screened? To a large extent the answer depends on how good the test is—in other words, is it accurate? Are there few false positives and few false negatives? Harm occurs in this case mainly when there are false positive tests, since the best evidence we have now suggests that a false negative test probably matters less because so many men die with prostate cancer than from prostate cancer. The false positive PSA test will certainly create anxiety, not only for the man but also for his family. Also, false positives are costly because in order to be certain that the result is a false positive, additional tests, including ultrasound studies and biopsies, are required.

If follow-up tests confirm prostate cancer, is there harm (besides costs) from treatment? Nearly eight per cent of men older than sixty-five years suffer from postoperative complications of the lungs or heart after their prostate cancer surgery. One per cent of these men die shortly after prostate surgery; in men older than seventy-four, the figure is two per cent. Surgery impairs sexual function in about fifty per cent and some degree of bladder control problem occurs in twenty-five per cent.[4] One study states, "...many patients and their physicians overestimate the likelihood of getting prostate cancer, dying from it, and receiving benefits from early detection and treatment. They underestimate the risks associated with early detection and intervention. These reported practice patterns and treatment beliefs may be due to aggressive marketing of early detection and treatment as rational, ethical, economical, effective, and necessary. The resulting epidemic of routine PSA testing regardless of age, medical condition, or scientific evidence has created a generation of patients, families, physicians, and media focused on PSA values."[5]

Why is there an "epidemic" of routine PSA testing when there is not yet good evidence that early diagnosis and treatment of prostate cancer makes a significant difference? The main reason is that many physicians and the public have been led to believe that doing the PSA for men who are older than fifty and without symptoms is a good idea. The widespread belief in the value of the test was based on early publications in reputable medical journals starting in the 1980s. There has been considerable controversy amongst doctors, however. By 1989, the U.S. Preventive Services Task Force (USPSTF), evaluating the evidence as outlined in this chapter, recommended against any routine screening for prostate cancer.[6]

In 1994, the Canadian Task Force on the Periodic Health Examination arrived at the same conclusion: "There is insufficient evidence to include prostate-specific antigen (PSA) screenings in the periodic health examination of men over fifty years of age. Exclusion is recommended on the basis of low positive value and the known risk of adverse effects associated with therapies of unproven effectiveness."[7] On the other hand, the American Cancer Society and the American Urological Association both recommended annual PSA testing in combination with a digital rectal examination for early detection of prostate cancer in men older than fifty years.[8] As of August 2006, the websites of both groups state that screening for prostate cancer should be offered to all men over fifty years and other men at high risk.

The reason for the differences in recommendations has to do with the manner in which the treatment guidelines are developed (see Chapter 10). Both U.S. and Canadian task forces use the approach outlined in this chapter, which means giving the most positive evaluations to research based on good studies, like RCTs when available, and the least value to the consensus arrived at by authorities in the field. Physicians in primary care (general practitioners and family physicians) have been trained by authorities, such as cancer specialists and urologists. When consensus is arrived at by groups such as the American Cancer Society and the American Urological Association, primary-care physicians tend to trust them and follow their guidelines. The practice of evidence-based medicine (EBM), defined as "the integration of our clinical expertise and our patients' values with the best available research evidence," is gaining popularity but has not yet completely replaced the practice of medicine based on advice from authorities. The best evidence includes clinically relevant research, often from the basic sciences of medicine, but especially from patient-centred clinical research into the accuracy and precision of diagnostic tests, the power of prognostic markers, and the efficacy and safety of therapeutic, rehabilitative and preventive interventions.[9] "Without this evidence, clinical practice risks becoming rapidly out of date, to our patients' detriment."[10]

So what should our healthy, fifty-year-old male do when his doctor recommends the PSA? The best answer is: wait. Fortunately, in 1995 a European randomized study of screening for prostate cancer involving 180,000 men—who were randomly allocated to be screened or not—was started. The objectives of the study are: to determine whether the effect of screening lowers the death rate of prostate cancer by at least twenty per cent; to identify the best screening method by selecting the most appropriate combination of available screening tests (PSA alone or combined with a rectal exam); to identify risk groups who will benefit most from the screening process; and to evaluate the quality of life of the participants and the cost-effectiveness of the screening program.[11]

The results of this study are expected by the year 2007. It is likely that results from this research will be able to answer this important question one way or the other.

There are many different types of screening tests. Here are a few that you might encounter; the list is by no means comprehensive.

Prenatal Ultrasounds

Challenge
Janet and her husband are delighted to learn that she is pregnant. Her physician recommends an ultrasound in the second trimester of pregnancy to determine if the fetus is normal and growing well. Janet realizes that if a serious abnormality in the fetus is found an abortion will be recommended.

Evidence
Randomized controlled trials have shown that early prenatal ultrasounds result in early detection of twins, a lower rate of induced labour, higher birth weights in singletons, and increased rates of abortion for fetal abnormalities.

Recommendation
An ultrasound in the second trimester is recommended.[12]

Challenge
The first ultrasound is completely normal. Janet continues to feel well and the doctor's examination concurs. She is told that further ultrasounds should be done in the second or third trimesters.

Evidence
Randomized controlled trials of serial ultrasounds have not shown any significant effects of pregnancy outcomes.

Recommendation

There is little evidence that further ultrasounds, after the first one is normal, should or should not be done. Thus, unless new studies find that the benefit exceeds the risks, they should not be done.

Screening for cervical cancer

Challenge

You are a healthy thirty-seven-year-old married woman with two children. Your family has recently moved to a new community and your new doctor does not recommend yearly screening for cervical cancer. Up until now you have been tested every year since you became sexually active at age eighteen and have found these tests very reassuring. Who is right: your previous doctor or your new doctor?

This dilemma is common, not only for patients but also for their physicians. A recent study has shown that seventy-five per cent of women studied preferred to be screened every year.[13] Sixty-nine per cent stated that they would seek yearly screening, even if their doctor informed them that less frequent screening had equally good results. In another study, obstetrician/gynecologists were surveyed about their cervical cancer screening practices. Three-quarters would begin screening virginal girls at eighteen years of age; sixty per cent would recommend annual screening in women even after three or more normal annual tests.[14]

Evidence

One of the problems is that early changes in the cervix suggestive of cancer may not progress to full-blown cancer, even without treatment. Nevertheless, there is evidence that screening works: there have been both cohort and case-control studies showing that women who are screened are much less likely to develop invasive cervical cancer. It has been estimated that because early changes progress to active cancer very slowly, screening every ten years would reduce serious disease by sixty-six per cent.[15]

Recommendation

Screening works. But how often should you be screened? It looks as though your new doctor is right. There is consensus that most women should be screened every three years once they have had normal readings from two consecutive annual tests. Testing should start with sexual activity or age eighteen. After two normal tests screening should be done every three years to age sixty-nine.[16]

Colorectal cancer

Challenge

Now that you, a very healthy fifty-one-year-old male with no family history of colorectal cancer, have gone in to see your doctor for a regular checkup, you are surprised that she has recommended colonoscopy screening. You are concerned that colonoscopy requires sedation because it can be painful, and the idea of a tube being placed high into your large intestine is scary. Last year you were screened with a test of your stool sample, which was negative for blood, making the risk of colorectal cancer quite low. It was a simple, painless, inexpensive test, and it reassured both you and your doctor. Your doctor wants to refer you for colonoscopy because recently the American College of Gastroenterology and the American Cancer Society have recommended colonoscopy every ten years for people of average risk beginning at age fifty.[17]

Evidence

There have been a number of randomized controlled trials showing that patients screened with the stool blood test have a lower risk of dying from colorectal cancer than unscreened patients. Testing yearly after age fifty leads to a greater reduction in mortality from colorectal cancer than testing every two years.[18]

As to the recommendations by prestigious authorities that colonoscopy should be added to low-risk groups as a screening procedure, both the U.S. Agency for Health Care Policy and Research and the U.S. Preventive Services Task Force agree that while colonoscopy is the most accurate test for detecting colorectal cancer, it is associated with higher risks for bleeding and perforation of the intestine and requires overnight bowel preparation, sedation, and a recovery time which may necessitate transportation for the patient. It is also much more expensive.

To summarize the evidence produced by these agencies: "No studies to date have been completed that show mortality reduction associated with screening colonoscopy,"[19] and "The USPSTF did not find direct evidence that screening colonoscopy is effective in reducing colorectal cancer mortality."[20]

Recommendation

The best advice would be to let your physician know that you would be happy to have a colonoscopy screening—once there is evidence from good studies which shows that the benefits outweigh the discomforts and risks. Until then, annual stool testing for blood would be your choice.

Cholesterol Screening

Challenge

You are a healthy, thirty-three-year-old woman of average weight; you do not smoke and have normal blood pressure. You have no first-degree relatives who are known to have coronary heart disease, and you are physically active, jogging for thirty minutes at least three times a week. During your regular checkup, your doctor wants to take blood for a cholesterol-lipid profile. You hate having blood taken. You ask why this is necessary since you are aware that you are at low risk for coronary heart disease. The doctor responds that the Expert Panel on Detection, Evaluation, and Treatment of High Blood Cholesterol has recommended that all adults aged twenty or older have a fasting lipoprotein profile done every five years.[21] What should you do?

Evidence

There is no question that mortality from coronary heart disease has decreased significantly in the past forty years.

In an attempt to determine what has led to this decrease, researchers assessed three main factors: first, prevention of heart disease in the general population; second, improvements in the acute treatment of patients who have heart attacks; and third, treatments of those patients who may not have had heart attacks but are diagnosed as having coronary heart disease. The authors of this study have calculated that about twenty-five per cent of the decrease is due to prevention in the general population, and seventy-five per cent is due to better acute and long-term management of patients with coronary heart disease.[22]

With regard to whether or not you should be screened with a cholesterol-lipid blood test, the answer is not simple. There have been no randomized controlled trials showing that average or low-risk adults who are screened are better off than those who are not. There have, on the other hand, been a number of RCTs showing that patients with elevated blood lipids who are treated, even if they have no symptoms of coronary heart disease, have a lower risk of dying or developing symptomatic coronary heart disease.[23]

Recommendation

Other than your dislike of being stuck with a needle, what is the harm of being screened with a cholesterol-lipid test? For example, what if your blood test is slightly abnormal but not enough for you to require treatment—does being labelled in this way produce anxiety or depression? This has been studied and has not been found to be a significant risk.[24]

So, again, what should you do? There is no evidence from RCTs that average to low-risk patients do better when screened than patients who are not screened. There is, however, good evidence that patients with risk factors who are treated do better. As you are healthy and have no first-degree relatives (male or female) with coronary heart disease (CHD), your risk of CHD is so low that screening is not indicated.

In summary, when good research studies show that screened patients live better, longer lives than do matched unscreened controls, those screening tests should be done. Fortunately more good research on screening tests is being done. Where the research has not been done, or the evidence is inconclusive, the risks may outweigh the benefits.[25]

References:

[1.] Kosters, J.P., Gotzsche, P.C., "CDC03373. Regular self-examination or clinical examination for early detection of breast cancer." Cochrane Database of Systematic Reviews, (2) 2003

[2.] Feightner, J.W., "Screening for Prostate Cancer." *The Canadian Guide to Clinical Preventive Health Care*, Canada Communication Group—Publishing, 813, 1994

[3.] Sandblom, G., Varenhorst, E., Lofman, O., et al. "Clinical consequences of screening for prostate cancer: 15 years follow-up of a randomized controlled trial in Sweden." *Eur Urol.*, 46(6): 717–23, 2004

[4.] Wilt, T.J. "Prostate Cancer Screening: Practice What the Evidence Preaches." *American Journal of Medicine* (AJM), 104: 602–604, 1998

[5.] Ibid.

6. U.S. Preventive Services Task Force, *Guide to Clinical Preventive Services.* Baltimore, MD: Williams & Wilkins; 1989

7. Ibid.

8. Meigs, J.B., Barry, M.J., Giovannuoci E., et al. "High Rates of Prostate-specific Antigen Testing in Men with Evidence of Benign Prostate Hyperplasia." *AJM*, 104: 517–525, 1998

9. Sackett, D.L., Rosenberg, W.M.C., Gray, J.A.M., et al. "Evidence-based medicine: what it is and what it isn't." *BMJ*, 312: 71–2, 1996

10. Straus, S.E., McAlister, F.A. "Evidence-Based Medicine: Past, Present, and Future." Annals RCPSC, 32:5, 260–264, 1999

11. Standaert, B., Denis, L. "The European Randomized Study of Screening for Prostate Cancer." *Cancer*, 80: 1830–1834, 1997

12. Anderson, G. "Routine Prenatal Ultrasound Screening." *The Canadian Guide to Clinical Preventive Health Care*, Canada Communication Group—Publishing, Ottawa, 4–14, 1994

13. Sirovich, B.E., Woloshin, S., Schwartz, L.M. "Screening for cervical cancer: will women accept less?" *AJM*, 118(2): 151–8, 2005

14. Saint, M,, Gildengorin, G., Sawaya, G.F. "Current cervical neoplasia screening practices of obstetrician/gynecologists in the US." *American Journal of Obstetrics and Gynecology*, 192(2): 414–21, 2005

15. Morrison, B.J. "Screening for cervical cancer." *The Canadian Guide To Clinical Preventive Health Care*, Canada Communication Group—Publishing, Ottawa, 884–889, 1994

16. Ibid.

17. Ransohoff, D.F., Sandler, R.S. "Screening for Colorectal Cancer." *New England Journal of Medicine* (NEJM), Vol.346, No.1, 40–44, 2002

18. Ibid.

19. "Colorectal Cancer Screening Summary, Evidence Report: Number 1." AHCPR Publication No.97-0302. Agency for Health Care Policy and Research, Rockville, MD. http://www.ahrq.gov/clinic/colorsum.htm

20. "Recommendations and Rationale: Screening for colorectal cancer," U.S. Preventive Services Task Force (USPSTF) (e-mail) ahrqpubs@hrq.gov

21. "Executive summary of the Third Report of the National Cholesterol Education Program (NCEP) Expert Panel on Detection, Evaluation, and Treatment of High Blood cholesterol in Adults (Adult Treatment Panel III)." *JAMA* 285; 2486–97, No.19, 2001

22. Goldman, Lee. Editorial: "The Decline in Coronary Heart Disease: Determining the Paternity of Success." *AJM*, 117:274–276, 2004

23. "Lipids and the Primary Prevention of Coronary Heart Disease: a National Clinical Guideline." Scottish Intercollegiate Guidelines Network. www.sign.ac.uk, 1999

24. Logan, A.G. "Lowering the Blood Total Cholesterol Level to Prevent Coronary Heart Disease." *Canadian Guide to Clinical Preventive Health Care*, Canada Communication Group— Publishing, Ottawa, 652–653, 1994

25. Feldman, W. "How Serious Are the Adverse Effects of Screening?" *Journal of General Internal Medicine*, 5(5 Suppl): 550–3, 1990

CHAPTER 5

When You Are Ill:
Are Tests Always Necessary?

Tests, when used appropriately, can speed up and confirm a diagnosis so that an effective treatment can begin earlier. This may not only make the patient feel better sooner by curing or alleviating a disease, but it may also save the patient (and the taxpayer) considerable amounts of money. A properly done test can shorten or avoid hospitalization, prevent the discomfort and costs of other tests, and may demonstrate that expensive medications are unnecessary.

Challenge: The Sore Throat

You are an eighteen-year-old university student, living away from home for the first time. For the last one and a half days, you've had a sore throat, fever, lack of appetite, and no energy. The doctor in the university health centre examines your throat, tells you that you have a streptococcal infection (strep throat) and is about to prescribe an antibiotic. You remember that the last time you had strep throat, your regular family doctor took a throat swab—a test to make sure it was the strep bacteria causing your ill-ness—before giving you an antibiotic. Your regular doctor felt that antibiotics were being over-prescribed for sore throats and that excessive use of antibiotics was the reason that many bacteria were becoming resistant to medication.

You tell the health centre doctor you would rather have a throat swab before you take antibiotics. He replies that you have all the clinical features that make him fairly cer-tain that it is strep and not an ordinary virus causing your illness and that a throat swab is unnecessary.

Who is right?

It is true that antibiotics have been over-prescribed and that this is a main cause for bacterial resistance. The real question is whether the doctor can accurately diagnose strep without the test, just by what is found in the his-tory of your illness and during the physical examination.

The strep throat swab is actually an excellent test—in fact, if done properly it is the "gold standard" to prove that strep is the cause of your illness. But is it necessary? The answer depends on how effectively the history and physical exam can act as a substitute for the lab test. Can a physician cut down the unnecessary use of antibiotics without doing a throat swab and not miss real cases of strep throat?

Fortunately there is good evidence that when certain criteria are used the accuracy of the diagnosis is excel-lent, even without the test. In fact, in one research study the examination by the doctor was evaluated in the way "tests" are evaluated, comparing the accuracy of the doc-

TAKE CONTROL OF YOUR HEALTH

tor's assessment with the gold standard, in this case, the throat swab. The doctor assigns one point for each of the following: fever equal to or greater than 38°C (100.04°F); absence of a cough; tender lymph glands in the neck; swelling or pus on the tonsils; and age less than fifteen years. If the patient is forty-five or older, one point is subtracted. If the score is one or less, neither a throat swab nor antibiotic therapy are needed. For a score of two or three, a throat swab is indicated and antibiotics given if the swab is positive for strep. Patients with a score of four or more have the highest likelihood of disease caused by strep and could either be given an antibiotic or a throat swab.[1]

In the study above the gold standard of the throat swab was done for all patients and compared with the score based on the doctors' assessments. The doctors were correct in almost all cases, diagnosing strep throat clinically eighty-five per cent of the time when it was actually there (sensitivity, or true positive) and diagnosing the sore throat as not being strep over ninety per cent of the time accurately (specificity, or true negative). This was true of patients treated by community-based family doctors as well as by doctors in a university-based family practice setting.

Does it matter if this scoring system misses ten per cent of the people with strep throat, or over-diagnoses strep throat in about fifteen per cent? Probably not. The missed ten per cent will either defeat the bacteria with their own immune system, or if they don't improve in a few days or get worse, will get treated. Similarly, over-diagnosing fifteen per cent is not a major problem. In fact, using the scoring system was shown to reduce over-all antibiotic prescription by over fifty per cent and to have reduced throat swabs by more than one-third.[2]

Therefore, as the eighteen-year-old with a fever of over 38°C (100.04°F), no cough, very tender neck glands, and swollen tonsils full of pus, you have scored four points and in all likelihood, you have strep throat. The health centre doctor, using this scoring system, felt that if you started antibiotics right away you would be able to get back to your classes earlier. On the other hand, he answered that if you would rather have the test and await the results before taking the antibiotics, he would be happy to do that.

You chose not to wait, took the antibiotic, felt much better by next morning and were back in class for your 10 a.m. lecture.

Challenge: The Sprained Ankle

Dorothy is a forty-year-old computer programmer who plays basketball with her friends on a weekly basis. During a recent game, she landed badly after jumping for a rebound and hurt her ankle. She limped over to the bench and, not wanting to stop the game, asked a teammate to replace her. Her plan was to rest for a while, then go home, wrap her ankle with an ice pack, and elevate her leg. Her teammate, Ellen, told her that she would drive her to the emergency room because when this had happened to her several weeks ago, the ER doctor told her that the only way to be sure there was no fracture was to x-ray the ankle.

When they got to the hospital, the ER doctor examined Dorothy's ankle, asked her to walk a few steps and told her there was no fracture. It was a sprain and she would be fine in a few days. At this point Ellen mentioned to the ER doctor what another doctor in the same hospital had told her about needing an x-ray.

Who is right?

There is good evidence that the doctor who told Dorothy she did not need an ankle x-ray was correct.

In a number of studies, doctors in Ottawa developed the Ottawa Ankle Rules, a list of criteria based on the doctor's examination, which correlate extremely well with the gold standard, the ankle x-ray. They showed that if the patient could bear weight on the ankle, even with a limp, both at the time of the injury and also later in the ER, the likelihood of a fracture was extremely low. When combined with the ankle examination done by the doctor, the Ottawa Ankle Rules put patients at virtually no risk of having a fracture undiagnosed. In the studies done in Ottawa, all patients—many hundreds—had an ankle x-ray done to see whether any fractures had been missed; none were missed. They showed that far fewer x-rays needed to be done after an ankle injury.[3] A recent review of thirty-two studies done in many countries confirmed the value of the Ottawa Ankle Rules as accurate and that fewer ankle x-rays were necessary when doctors used the rules.[4]

In this chapter, I have described two situations where there is good evidence that a careful assessment by the doctor may make a test—either a lab test (throat swab

for strep throat) or an x-ray (ankle x-ray for a sprain)—
unnecessary. In the next chapter I describe the ideal
properties of tests that may be necessary for the doctor
to make a diagnosis when you are ill.

References:

[1.] McIssac, W.J., Goel, V., To, T., and Low, D. "The validity of a
sore throat score in family practice." *CMAJ* , 163(7): 811–5, 2000

[2.] Ibid.

[3.] Strell, I.G., Greenberg, H.H., Mc Knight, R.D., et al. "Decision
Rules for the Use of Radiography in Acute Ankle Injuries:
Refinement and Prospective Validation." *JAMA,* 269: 1127–1132,
1993

[4.] Bachmann, L.M., Kolb, E., Koller, M.T., et al. "Accuracy of
Ottawa ankle rules to exclude fractures of the ankle and mid-
foot: systematic review." *BMJ*, Feb.22; 326(7386), 417, 2003

CHAPTER 6

Making the Diagnosis

Webster's Dictionary defines diagnosis as "the discrimination of diseases by their distinctive marks or symptoms; the examination of a person to discover what ailment affects him." In the previous chapter two diagnoses— strep throat and sprained ankle—were made without the use of any lab tests or x-rays.

A correct diagnosis is crucial and is the foundation upon which the prognosis and treatment depend. Prognosis is defined as a prediction or conclusion regarding the course of a disease and the probability of recovery. Before the physician and patient make the decision about treatment and how it will affect the course of the disease they need to be certain that the diagnosis is correct.

In this chapter the steps taken to make a diagnosis and the properties of tests that may be necessary during this process are discussed.

Challenge 1

Your four-year-old daughter complains for the first time that she has pain when she urinates. She is urinating more frequently than usual and she is beginning to cry each time. Her doctor examines her, checks her urine, and confirms that, as you suspected, she has a urinary tract infection. He prescribes an antibiotic and by the next day she is much better. When you call his office to let him know of her improvement, as he had asked you to do, he says he will book an appointment for her to have some tests in the x-ray department in about one month. When you tell him that you yourself have had several urinary tract infections and were not advised to have kidney or bladder x-rays, he says that these tests are commonly done on children to make sure that their kidneys, ureters, and bladder are normal. Some children are born with blockages or leaks in the urinary tract and may need corrective surgery to prevent serious kidney damage.

What should you do?

The first question to be answered is: what is the evidence that children like your daughter benefit from these tests? Your daughter has been very healthy, had her first urinary tract infection when she was four years old, and responded very well to treatment. Most of the studies showing blockages or leaks in the urinary system using a variety of tests in the x-ray departments were done in children who were *not* like your daughter. Most of them were from major university hospitals where sicker children tend to be cared for. They tend to have had their first infections before they were two years old, and were often quite sick with these infections and had high fevers. Many of them were boys. In other words, these studies suffered from an important bias called the "referral bias," which means the tests were done on the sickest children who were referred to specialists whose patients were different than the average; they were referred because their own doctors had trouble looking after their illnesses. They were likelier to have been born with structural problems in their genitourinary (parts of the body that play a role in reproduction or getting rid of urine, or both) system.

What is quite common in the genitourinary tracts of children with urinary tract infections is a condition called vesicoureteral reflux (VUR), which is a leak from the bladder back into the tubes coming from the kidneys—the ureters. Most of the time this leak is not severe. At one time it was believed that significant VUR on both sides required surgery to prevent kidney damage. This is the basis for the diligence with which doctors have looked for VUR. Fortunately, a randomized controlled trial in which children with severe VUR were either operated on or treated medically has shown no better results ten years later in the children operated on—the changes in kidney function were minimal and were the same in both groups.[1] In another study children treated without surgery actually improved. They had less VUR five years later and even better results at ten years.[2]

In our example, tests of the urine sample confirmed an infection: the diagnosis was important because there is effective treatment. In otherwise healthy four-year-old girls like the patient presented, is it important to make a diagnosis of VUR? If there is no good evidence that surgery will make a difference even if the reflux is diagnosed, why are further tests in the x-ray department necessary?

In fact, for otherwise healthy four-year-olds with their first uncomplicated urinary tract infection there is little evidence that routine imaging (tests done in the x-ray department) improves outcomes.[3] While there is no evidence of benefit from making the diagnosis of VUR in this patient, there is the potential of harm. If she is found to have VUR which does not require treatment, there may be considerable anxiety within the family because "she has something wrong with her kidneys."

Because there is little evidence that making a diagnosis of VUR in your daughter would be of benefit, she does not need to have any studies in the x-ray department at this time. Should she have recurrent urinary tract infections or infections in which she looks more ill than she did with this one, or if subsequent infections do not respond as well to treatment, then further tests in the x-ray department may be indicated. In this example, the urine tests confirming the infection are necessary; the tests to diagnose VUR are not.

How do doctors make a diagnosis?

Each illness is associated with symptoms—feelings that the patients themselves have noticed—and signs—findings discovered by the physician during the physical examination.

The best description of the act of making a diagnosis is the following: "The act of clinical diagnosis is classification for a purpose: an effort to recognize the class or group to which a patient's illness belongs so that, based on [the physician's] prior experience with that class, the subsequent clinical acts we can afford to carry out, and the patient is willing to follow, will maximize that patient's health."[4]

A common approach used by physicians is "pattern recognition." For example, when skin lesions are so characteristic of a skin disorder the physician has seen many times before, the diagnosis is easy.

When the diagnosis is not so obvious the physician asks a series of questions and organizes the questioning and components of the physical examination in a branching manner.

Challenge 2

Dan, a sixty-year-old accountant, has been brought to the emergency room with severe chest pain and shortness of breath. He has never experienced this before.

The staff in the ER realize that Dan is quite ill and see him immediately. The strategy used by the nurses and doctors in making the diagnosis of Dan's illness is described as follows: "It is the formulation, from the earliest clues about the patient, of a short list of potential diagnoses or actions, followed by the performance of those clinical (history and physical exam) and paraclinical (e.g. laboratory, x-ray) manoeuvres that will best reduce the length of the list."[5] The short list uses diagnostic labels (in Dan's case, heart attack, blood clot in the lung, etc.) as a way of understanding the biological changes that could explain the illness.

Doctors use their experience to shorten the list of possible diagnoses by taking a focused history, doing a physical examination, and doing (hopefully) the smallest number of laboratory tests required to make the diagnosis. There are three main reasons why unnecessary tests should be avoided. First, not all tests are one hundred per cent accurate and a false positive test can produce anxiety. Second, the false positive test will require additional and repeat tests to determine whether it was accurate, leading to additional time, discomfort, and anxiety. And finally, tests are often expensive. Thus only those tests required to confirm or negate the suspected diagnosis should be done.

In the previous chapter there was good evidence that in many cases patients with acute sore throats or sprained ankles receive appropriate treatment even when no tests are done.

In Dan's case, a possible heart attack, certain tests are necessary for two reasons: first, a correct diagnosis made within a short period of time could save his life, and second, there are tests which can give the correct diagnosis in minutes.

The death rate from heart attacks has dropped more than fifty per cent in the past thirty years.[6] A significant cause of this mortality decrease is better management in the first few hours and days.[7] A key component in making the diagnosis of a heart attack is the electrocardiogram (EKG), which can help determine the intensity and speed of care required when a patient is admitted with a heart attack. The two main causes of death shortly after a heart attack are 1) when so much heart muscle is damaged that the heart no longer works well as a pump, leading to heart failure, and 2) the location of the damage. In other words the amount of damage may be small but it may be in a location required for the heart to beat in a regular rhythm—abnormalities in the rhythm can also lead to heart failure and death. Researchers who evaluate exactly how useful a test is ask a number of questions.

Was the test ever studied and compared to a gold standard?

In the case of the EKG, the answer is yes. The gold standard in this case is the pathologist's autopsy report. In the past thirty years, the mortality rate and the autopsy rate have both decreased, however, so the EKG abnormalities shown in patients who died of heart attacks in previous years have become well recognized. Blood tests which demonstrate heart muscle damage are valuable in those few cases where the EKG changes are not striking. Also, some patients with chest pain may have a normal initial EKG but when the test is redone a few days later the results could be abnormal.

Positive predictive value is defined as the proportion of patients with abnormal test results who have the disease for which they were tested. It is known that eighty per cent of heart attacks affect the right coronary artery and the positive predictive value of certain EKG changes for such a heart attack is one hundred per cent.[8] Thus, one hundred per cent of patients with certain changes in the EKG have heart attacks involving the right coronary artery.

What about patients with EKGs showing no evidence of changes due to right coronary artery blockage? The negative predictive value, i.e. the proportion of patients with negative tests results who do not have the disease, in this case is eighty-eight per cent.[9]

Should one be concerned about the observation that twelve per cent of patients with initial EKGs not showing right coronary artery changes may have had a heart attack which may be missed? Not really, because other factors—the blood test showing heart muscle destruction, or repeat EKGs which become abnormal over the next few days—will confirm the diagnosis.

Are patients in the study similar?

Is the setting of the research similar to the ER where Dan was seen? In the case of the EKG, which has been around for many years, it has been used in many patients with chest pain and shortness of breath like Dan's, in doctors' offices, in emergency rooms and coronary care units, as well as in ambulances. In one study EKGs done in the ambulance were found to be very predictive of heart attacks.[10]

Is the test objective and accurate?

For example, if an EKG result were shown to two separate doctors would they interpret the results in the same way? This is called inter-observer variability. If one were to show the same EKG to the same doctor at two different times, how often would the physician agree with his/her previous interpretation? This is known as intra-observer variability. For example in a study that performed exercise EKGs in patients who were *not* having heart attacks but who might have underlying problems with their coronary arteries, two cardiologists interpreted the results in the same way only fifty-seven per cent of the time. When one cardiologist reviewed the same exercise EKGs at two separate times, the agreement was only seventy-four per cent.

Fortunately this is not the case for patients suspected of having heart attacks. Agreement was very high amongst a variety of doctors but highest when the EKGs were read by the most highly trained in this area, cardiologists.[11]

Finally, the last question one should ask regarding a lab test has to do with the definition of "abnormal."

Challenge 3

James, a thirty-five-year-old mechanic, is scheduled to have an elective operation for a hernia. The day before the surgery, a number of blood tests are performed in the hospital where the surgery will be done. The operation may be cancelled if the fasting blood sugar is elevated. The normal upper level for fasting blood sugar in that hospital is 140 mg/dl (7.8 mmol/L). James' level was found to be 148.

Does this mean that James could have diabetes? How "abnormal" is 148? The answer depends on a number of factors. First, James has no symptoms of diabetes: excessive thirst, frequency of urinating large volumes, waking up at night to drink and to urinate. He is fit, not overweight, and has no family history of diabetes.

Secondly, in the absence of any symptoms of illness, 148 may merely be a statistic. The definition of abnormal (for most blood tests) is made by checking many healthy persons and ranking the lowest 2.5 per cent as "abnormally" low, and the highest 2.5 per cent as too high. Thus anybody, including healthy people, has a five per cent chance of having an "abnormal" test: too high or too low.

James insists on having another fasting blood sugar. The surgeon agrees—the result is 136 and the surgery is successfully completed.

In summary, when making a diagnosis, the physician relies mainly on the patients' symptoms and the physical examination. When tests are needed, they should have good evidence of scientific validity and of value in helping the patient.

References:

[1.] Smellie, J.M., Barratt, T.M., Chantler, C., et al. "Medical versus surgical treatment in children with severe bilateral reflux and bilateral nephropathy: a randomized trial." *The Lancet,* 357: 1329–33, 2001

[2.] Smellie, J.M., Jodal, U., Lax, H., et al. "Outcome at 10 years of severe vesicoureteral reflux managed medically: report of the international reflux study in children." *Journal of Pediatrics,* 139: 656–63, 2001

3. Dick, P.T. "Urinary Tract Problems in Primary Care." *Evidence-Based Pediatrics,"* W. Feldman, editor, B.C. Decker Inc., Hamilton, London, Saint Louis, 2000

4. Sackett, D.L., Haynes, R.B., Guyatt, G., and Tugwell, P. *Clinical Epidemiology: A Basic Science for Clinical Medicine, 2nd Edition.* Little, Brown and Company, Boston, Toronto, London, 1991

5. Ibid.

6. Levy, D., Thom, T. Editorial: "Death Rates from Coronary Disease—Progress and a Paradox." *NEJM,* 339:13, 915–917, 1998

7. Rosamond, W.D., Chambless, L.E., Folsom, A.R. et al. "Trends in the Incidence of Myocardial Infarction and in Mortality Due to Coronary Heart Disease, 1987 to 1994." *NEJM,* 339:861–7, 1998

8. Zimetbaum, P.J., Josephson, M.D. "Use of the electrocardiogram in acute myocardial infarction." *NEJM,* 348:10, 933–940, 2003

9. Ibid.

10. Svenson, L., Axelsson, C., Nordlander, R., et al. "Prehospital identification of acute coronary syndrome/myocardial infarction in relation to ST elevation." *International Journal of Cardiology* 98: (2), 237–244, 2005

11. Mensel, D. "Observer variability in ECG interpretation for thrombolysis eligibility: experience and context matter." *Journal of Thrombosis and Thrombolysis,* 15(3): 131–40, 2003

CHAPTER 7

The Importance of a
Correct Prognosis

Prognosis is defined as a prediction or conclusion regarding the course of a disease and the probability of recovery. Knowing the course of a disease is important for the patient as well as the family. The importance of prognosis is paramount in much decision-making, whether it is in the doctor's office, the emergency room, or the intensive care unit—in short, whenever a patient is ill.

Challenge

You notice that Sally, your eighteen-month-old daughter, is a bit cranky. She has had a cold for a few days. She has not eaten much for supper. You are getting her ready for bed and notice that she feels hot. You take her temperature and it is 39°C (102.2°F). Just after you give her some anti-fever medication she has a convulsion. She loses consciousness and has twitching movements in her arms and legs. You rush her to the emergency department. Although you were very frightened and worried that she might die, you did notice that the convulsion lasted about seven minutes and is over by the time she is seen by the ER doctor. She now actually looks reasonably well, and by the time her temperature is taken in the ER, about forty-five minutes after the anti-fever medication, it is down to 38°C (100.02°F).

After a thorough examination, the doctor tells you that Sally has had a febrile convulsion, a benign condition that some children get when they have a high fever. You and your spouse have many questions, not so much about the diagnosis because Sally looks really well again, but about the future: will she have more of these attacks? Could she go on to have epilepsy? Could febrile convulsions affect her mental development? If they do recur, will she outgrow them? When? What about her two-month-old brother? How can we prevent recurrences?

Will she have more febrile seizures?

In order to answer this question, it is important to note that there are two kinds of febrile seizures, simple and complex.[1] The prognosis is different for each of these categories. Sally's seizure is likely in the "simple" class, because both sides of her body were twitching, the episode lasted less than ten minutes and stopped without anticonvulsant therapy. If she has no further convulsions in the next twenty-four hours, the diagnosis of simple febrile seizure will be confirmed. The definition of complex febrile seizure requires the seizure to recur within twenty-four hours, involves just one side of the body, or lasts more than ten minutes.

One of the problems in answering your questions about Sally is that many of the studies about the prognosis of this condition lump simple and complex seizures together. Thus it is important to assess in a study on prognosis whether the patients being followed are similar to your child. For example, to answer your question about whether Sally will have more seizures next time she gets a fever, one has to ascertain from the research a) whether the patients followed all had simple febrile seizures and b) whether there may have been a referral bias, which there may be if the cases are reported from a pediatric neurology clinic (these are more serious cases that family doctors and general pediatricians referred because they were hard to manage) and not from the community. In one review of fourteen research papers on the prognosis of febrile seizures, the risk of recurrence varied from twenty-nine per cent to fifty-five per cent, with the higher risks reported from clinic-based as opposed to community-based studies.[2]

The recurrence rate for febrile seizures is greater if the following characteristics are present: the first seizure occurred when the child was younger than fourteen months; the fever was not very high at the time of the seizure; the child had a very short illness before the seizure; and a family history of febrile seizures is present. If all four of these are present, the risk of recurrence is about eighty per cent. If there are no risk factors, the risk of another febrile seizure before the child has outgrown the risk is only around ten to fifteen per cent.[3]

What about the chances of your child developing epilepsy?

Most experts agree that the risk of developing epilepsy for most children with a simple febrile seizure is not much greater than the risk of epilepsy in the general population: between two and four per cent.[4] However, one review of five studies of large samples of children followed after their first febrile seizure showed differences in the proportions who went on to have epilepsy as low as two per cent to as high as ten per cent.[5] Risk factors for epilepsy following a febrile seizure include: a seizure involving only one side of the body; the initial seizure lasting more than ten minutes; two or more seizures within the same illness that causes the fever; the child being developmentally delayed at the time of the seizure; and a family history of epilepsy. Your child has none of these characteristics and therefore her likelihood of developing epilepsy is about the same as if she had not had the seizure. If she had several of these factors, her risk of epilepsy would be ten to fifteen per cent.[6,7] In other words, in order to get an accurate prediction as to how things will turn out, the research has to be done on patients very similar to the one under consideration.

Could febrile convulsions affect her mental development?

Up until the time of the seizure, Sally's development was, if anything, ahead of schedule. Because the quality of some of the studies varied, it was previously difficult to state with complete certainty that there is no effect on children's intelligence if they have a simple febrile convulsion, although most experts felt that the IQ and behaviour of these children was the same as that of their unaffected siblings.[8] In an attempt to overcome some of the methodological weakness of other studies, eighty children who had had febrile seizures were followed along with eighty-eight children who had not. Two years after the seizure, both groups were assessed using established behavioural and IQ tests—no differences were found.[9]

Will she outgrow the risk of recurrence? If so, at what age?

The National Institute of Health's (NIH) definition of febrile seizures includes an age range from three months to five years; thus, if she does not have another febrile seizure before she reaches five, there will not be a recurrence. In fact, even if she does have a recurrence before age five, the likelihood of recurrences thereafter is remote.

What about her two-month-old brother? Is he likely to have a seizure when he gets a fever?

There does seem to be an inherited predisposition to febrile seizures, even if neither parent had them as children. For example, if one identical twin has a febrile seizure, it is highly likely that the other twin will also have a seizure when s/he has a fever. However, if the twins are non-identical the likelihood is no greater than that of non-twin siblings. The risk of a febrile seizure for your son is between nine and seventeen per cent, which means there is a better than eighty per cent chance of his not having one.[10] In this condition as in others, in order to determine if there is an inherited tendency one should review studies comparing identical twins, who have the same genes, with non-identical twins. If the problem is seen more often in the identical twins, then one can be sure there is a genetic component to the condition.

How can we prevent recurrences?

The answer to this question is based on two factors: first, we now know that Sally's prognosis of being a healthy, normal child is based on sound evidence; even if she does have a recurrence, she will do fine. Second, we now know that although daily anticonvulsant medications may prevent recurrences, they may also do more harm than good. Daily anticonvulsant medication has been shown in randomized controlled trials in children with febrile seizures to cause behavioural and learning difficulties.[11]

To summarize, in order to have confidence in the prognosis of a condition one should be sure that the nature of the problem is very similar between the patient under consideration and those in the prognosis research study. In addition, the follow-up should be as long and complete as necessary to get a true picture of the future for the patient being considered.[12]

References

1. Wariuru, C., Appleton, R. "Febrile seizures: an update." *Archives of Disease in Childhood*, Aug 89(8): 751–6, 2004

2. Berg, A.T., Shinnar, S., Hauser, W.A., and Leventhal, J.M. "Predictors of recurrent febrile seizures: A meta-analytic review." *Journal of Pediatrics*, 116: 329–37, 1990

3. Camfield, P., Camfield, C. "Seizure Disorders." *Evidence-Based Pediatrics,* W. Feldman, editor, B.C. Decker, Hamilton London, St. Louis, p231, 2000

4. Ibid.

5. Shinnar, S., Glauser, T.A. "Febrile seizures." *Journal of Child Neurology*, Jan, 17 Suppl.: S44–52, 2002

6. Nelson, K., Ellenberg, J. "Prognosis in children with febrile seizures." *Pediatrics*, 61: 720–7, 1978

7. Annegers, J.F., Hauser, W.A., Shirts, S.B., et al. "Factors prognostic of unprovoked seizures after febrile convulsions." *NEJM*, 316: 493–8, 1987

8. Gordon, K.E., Dooley, J.M., Camfield, P.R., et al. "Treatment of febrile seizures: the influence of treatment efficacy and side-effect profile on value to parents." *Pediatrics,* Nov, 105(5): 1080–8, 2001

9. Kolfen, W., Pehle, K., Konig, S. "Is the long-term outcome of children following febrile convulsions favorable?" *Developmental Medicine and Child Neurology*, Oct; 40(10): 667–71, 1998

10. Fishman, M.A. "Febrile seizures." *Pediatrics*, A.M. Rudolph, editor, Appleton & Lange, 1987

11. Camfield, P., Camfield, C. "Seizure Disorders." *Evidence-Based Pediatrics,* W. Feldman, editor, B.C. Decker, Hamilton, London, St. Louis, p231, 2000

12. Laupacis, A., Wells, G., Richardson, W.S., et al. "Users guides to the medical literature. V. How to use an article about prognosis." *JAMA*, July 20, 272(3), 234–37, 1994

CHAPTER 8

Treatment: How to Make Sure that Treatment Does More Good than Harm

Society has given physicians and surgeons immense power to affect people's lives. The right to prescribe powerful medications, to perform surgery, or to recommend psychotherapy dealing with a patient's darkest secrets comes with the responsibility to be as certain as possible that the benefits of treatment outweigh the potential risks.

Challenge 1

Roberta, a fifty-two-year-old married chef, has recently been told that she has breast cancer. The tumour is one inch in diameter and there is no evidence that it has spread. The surgeon to whom she has been referred advises her that the safest form of therapy to prevent the cancer from spreading is to remove the whole breast with a mastectomy.

She and her husband are overwhelmed. They spend some time looking up breast cancer treatment on the Internet and read that a lumpectomy, which removes just the cancer and not the whole breast, has results that are just as good.

Who is right?

For many years, mastectomy was the treatment of choice. Because of the cosmetic problems associated with this surgery researchers began to ask whether lumpectomy, while making certain that there was no spread at the time of surgery, would have results as good as mastectomy without the disfigurement. Two groups of researchers, one in Italy[1] and another in the U.S.,[2] did randomized controlled trials in which women with relatively small breast cancers were treated with mastectomy or breast-conserving lumpectomy surgery. In the U.S. study some of the women undergoing lumpectomy were assigned to a group in which radiation therapy was added to the surgery.

Both groups of researchers followed their patients for twenty years. The baseline characteristics of the patients assigned to the various groups were similar with regard to age, onset of menopause, the size of the tumour and spread of the tumour to the lymph glands under the arm.

Twenty years later, thirty-seven per cent of the patients in the U.S. study were alive and cancer-free. The rates of survival in the three treatment groups (mastectomy, lumpectomy alone, lumpectomy plus irradiation) were not significantly different. In the Italian study, women had either mastectomy or lumpectomy plus radiation. The twenty-year survival rate was fifty-six per cent, similar in both groups.

Because fewer women who received lumpectomy plus radiation had a recurrence of cancer in the same breast, lumpectomy plus radiation and removal of the affected lymph glands has become the standard of care for women with breast tumours up to five centimetres.

The reason for the better twenty-year survival rate in the Italian study is that the tumours in the U.S. study were larger (up to four centimetres) compared with those in the Italian study (no larger than two centimetres).

In an editorial in the same journal in which the two studies were published, Dr. Monica Morrow reveals that even though there was evidence before these definitive studies were published that lumpectomy plus radiation was as effective as mastectomy many surgeons were still recommending mastectomy. She states, "It is time to declare the case against breast-conserving therapy closed...."[3]

Challenge 2

Albert, a sixty-one-year-old otherwise healthy pharmacist, has just been told he has prostate cancer. The urologist to whom he has been referred assures him that the tumour is small, has not spread, and that with surgery called radical prostatectomy, the prognosis is excellent. Albert asks about side effects following surgery and is told that there is a risk of bladder incontinence and/or of impotence.

Albert and his wife are both concerned about these complications of surgery and review material they find on the Internet. They find that "watchful waiting," in which the patients are followed carefully without surgery, has fewer bad side effects than prostatectomy and may have as good a prognosis regarding mortality.

What decision should Albert make?

The evidence required to help in such important decision-making is starting to become more solid. In one randomized controlled trial 695 men younger than seventy-five, with newly diagnosed prostate cancer in the early stages, were assigned to have either radical prostatectomy or watchful waiting.[4] The randomization was designed in a way to ensure that the groups would be as similar as possible before the study began: they were comparable in age, PSA level, tumour stage, and the method of detection of the cancer (screening, symptoms, etc.). Follow-up was done twice a year for two years, then once a year, for a median follow-up of 6.2 years. The health status of the patients in the follow-up was assessed by the study researchers in a blinded manner, which meant they were unaware as to whether the patients had been operated on or not. In reviewing the causes of death in those who died during the follow-up, the researchers were also blinded as to which group the patients had been assigned. If the autopsy reported that death was caused by prostate cancer, this was accepted as the cause. If the autopsy showed the patient died with prostate cancer but from another disease, e.g. a heart attack, the death was recorded as not due to prostate cancer.

The researchers were careful to select a large enough sample of patients so that the possibility of a difference of the outcomes between the two groups being due to chance rather than being a true difference was very unlikely. Similarly, the numbers were large enough to be quite certain that they would not miss a small but important difference between the groups.

In addition, they carefully recorded what treatment the patients actually received rather than merely to which group they had been assigned. The reason for this is that in this kind of research the subjects can change their minds after they had been assigned to a group and opt for the alternate approach. For example, twenty-five of the 347 men assigned to the radical prostatectomy group opted for watchful waiting, and twenty-three of the 348 men assigned to the watchful waiting group chose to have surgery.

The results were interesting: the death rates at 6.2 years follow-up were the same in both groups.

The same group of researchers, in another paper, reported on the complications of watchful waiting or radical prostatectomy.[5] They selected patients from the previously described study enrolled during a specified time period and from certain geographic areas. Questionnaires were mailed to about fifty per cent of the total sample, and a very high percentage responded— eighty-seven per cent. Although the patients in both groups felt their overall quality of life was similar, impotence was eighty per cent in the surgical group and only forty-five per cent in the watchful waiting group. Similarly, urinary leakage was more than twice as high in the prostatectomy group; forty-nine per cent versus twenty-one per cent in the watchful waiting group.

Ten years after the study began, the researchers did find a slight decrease in overall mortality for the prostatectomy group, but because side effects were so significant, the authors concluded that "…clinical decision-making and patient counselling will remain difficult."[6] In other words, given all the evidence, the patient should make the decision.

Let us review the key questions that need to be answered when making a decision about a treatment.

Are there any randomized controlled trials demonstrating that the treatment is effective and safe?

This should be the case not only for serious conditions like cancer but also for less serious conditions like the common cold in children. For example, although over-the-counter cold medications are extremely widely used, a review of controlled studies revealed that of more than one hundred such trials, only four had been done on children, and only two on preschool-aged children. Both of these studies showed no benefits in children randomized to take the medication compared with those taking placebos.[7]

How valid were the randomized controlled trials?

Was the selection process into one or another of the groups being studied (new treatment vs. traditional therapy or placebo) truly random? If the investigators know in advance to which group someone in the study will be assigned, they could, if they have a bias in favour of the treatment being studied, consciously or unconsciously enrol those subjects less seriously ill to the treatment group.

Were all the important outcomes necessary to assess benefits vs. harms studied and reported?

For example, in the prostate cancer study in which the overall quality of life status in the surgery group was similar to that of the watchful waiting group, it was important that the researchers found the differences in bladder control and impotence. These differences may be helpful in making the decision as to whether or not to have the surgery.

Were the patients in the trial similar to you?

If your breast cancer is small, then lumpectomy plus irradiation is what you would likely choose. If your child is two years old, over-the-counter cold medications won't help, but there is evidence that they do work in teenagers.

Is the sample size large enough so that differences in outcomes are unlikely to have occurred just by chance?

In other words, are there enough individuals enrolled in the study to ensure that if no differences were found, the lack of a difference is likely to be real and not a fluke?

Are identified differences between the treatments being studied vs. the traditional treatment or placebo really important?

For example, the new migraine medication might provide the treatment group one headache per month less than the placebo group, but produce more side effects like nausea. Patients may prefer the additional headache in order to avoid the risk of nausea.

Is the treatment available to you?

For example, if a new arthritis treatment can only be provided in highly specialized programs hundreds of miles away from where you live, can you afford the cost and time away from work or can you cope with the pain using traditional treatments?

Were all the patients who entered the trial accounted for at the end of the study?

Unless this is the case, the conclusions of the study may be invalid because some patients got better quickly and dropped out of the study, or died, possibly as a result of the new treatment or because they received the traditional therapy or a placebo. If these deaths and the causes of death are not accounted for, or the reasons for the dropouts are not uncovered, and if the patients not accounted for represent a significant number, the true benefits or harms of the treatment might be unclear.

In summary, patients who know what questions to ask their physicians when a treatment is recommended are likely to make decisions based on good evidence that the treatment will do more good than harm. Similarly, when seeking information in the media or on the Internet, patients who ask the right questions will make better decisions regarding their health.

References:

[1] Veronesi, U., Cascinelli, N., Mariani, L., et al. "Twenty-year follow-up of a randomized study comparing breast-conserving surgery with radical mastectomy for early breast cancer." *NEJM*, 347: 1227–32, 2002

[2] Fisher, B., Anderson, S., Bryant, J., et al. "Twenty-year follow-up of a randomized trial comparing total mastectomy, lumpectomy, and lumpectomy plus irradiation for the treatment of invasive breast cancer." *NEJM*, 347: 1233–41, 2002

[3] Morrow, M. Editorial. *NEJM*, 347, (16), 1270–1271, 2002

[4] Holmberg, L., Bill-Axelson, A., Helgesen, F., et al. "A Randomized trial comparing radical prostatectomy with watchful waiting in early prostate cancer." *NEJM*, 347: 781–9, 2002

[5] Steineck, G., Helgesen, F., Adolfsson, J., et al. "Quality of life after radical prostatectomy or watchful waiting." *NEJM*, 347: 790–6, 2002

[6] Bill-Axelson, A., Holmberg, L., Ruutu, M., et al. "Radical Prostatectomy versus Watchful Waiting in Early Prostate Cancer." *NEJM*, 352:1977–84, 2005

[7] Smith, M.B.H., Feldman, W., "Over-the-counter cold medications: A critical review of clinical trials between 1950 and 1991." *JAMA,* 269: 2258–2263, 1993

CHAPTER 9

Clinical Practice Guidelines: Can Patients Use Them?

Doctors are overwhelmed with medical information. There are more than four hundred thousand articles in medical journals every year. Obviously, these are not all relevant to the average physician—many articles deal with laboratory research and do not apply to a physician's daily practice. However, many are relevant. Because reading medical journals is how most doctors keep up-to-date, and because most doctors work more than fifty hours a week seeing patients, getting the best evidence-based information presents a challenge.

For these reasons, various groups have developed clinical practice guidelines.

Clinical practice guidelines are "systematically developed statements to assist practitioner and patient decisions about appropriate health care for specific clinical circumstances."[1]

Although many clinical practice guidelines (CPGs) have been written and published—the American Medical Association listed 2200 practice guidelines in

1997[2]—their uptake and use by doctors has not been particularly widespread.

One of the main reasons for the relatively low popularity of CPGs has to do with the phrase "systematically developed statements." Because not all CPGs are based on sound evidence, they may confuse physicians because of conflicting advice. For example, in 1997, within a short time, two groups published opposing recommendations on mammography for women under age fifty.[3,4]

For patients who wish to get sound evidence in caring for their health, CPGs can be very helpful if used properly.

Challenge

You are a forty-seven-year-old sales clerk who was found to have high blood pressure during your regular checkup. Your doctor checked your blood pressure several times on the first visit, and to be sure your pressure wasn't elevated because of anxiety about seeing the doctor (so called "white coat" syndrome) she asked you to come back again the next day. Again, the blood pressure was the same as the day before (145/95) and stayed the same after being taken several times over the next hour. You are not overweight and you are a non-smoker who exercises regularly. Because your late father had hypertension, (high blood pressure) you have been very careful about the amount of salt in your diet.

Your doctor recommends that you take an inexpensive generic medication that has been used for many years with good results. However, you found out from colleagues at work that there are newer antihypertensive medications, non-generic and more expensive, that work even better.

What should you do?

To be sure that the treatment you take is effective and safe, tell your doctor that you would like one day to think about it. You go home, go to your Internet search engine and type in "clinical practice guidelines for hypertension." There will be several, some put out by medical associations, universities, governments, government-funded organizations such as the U.S. National Institute of Health, and more.

Which ones should you look at first? There are guidelines published by groups without a conflict of interest (i.e. not funded by industries selling products such as pharmaceuticals and alternative health products). These groups generally (not only for hypertension) produce sound, evidence-based guidelines. These groups include the Agency for Health Care Policy and Research, the Canadian Task Force on Preventive Health Care, the U.S. Preventive Services Task Force, the Agency for Health Care Research and Quality the Institute for Clinical Systems Improvement, and the Scottish Intercollegiate Guidelines Network.

If any of these are listed in the topic you are looking for, read them first.

Second, check the year the guidelines were published. Even some of the best guidelines may be out of date because of new evidence. For example, a review of the guidelines produced by an excellent agency revealed that many were out of date. The authors concluded that "as a general rule, guidelines should be reassessed for validity every three years."[5] If one of the established guideline agencies listed above has a guideline that is more than three years old, try to find a more recent one put out by another agency on the list.

Next, make sure the guideline is written about patients like you. For example, aside from your hypertension, you and your physician agree that you are very healthy. Therefore guidelines written for hypertension in diabetics or patients with chronic kidney disease are not for you, nor are those written dealing with hypertension in patients with heart failure.

If you find an up-to-date guideline written for people like you, try to assess whether the guideline developers have a conflict of interest where they are funded by a drug company which may manufacture a drug for hypertension. Where guidelines differ, (as in chapter 5 regarding PSA screening for prostate cancer when the American Urological Association and the American Cancer Society recommending screening, whereas the U.S. Preventive Services Task Force and Canadian Task Force on Preventive Health Care concluded that the evidence to include PSA is not there) the judgment must be made on the quality of the evidence one way or the other.

The best way to assess whether there is a conflict of interest is to see whether there is a statement as to who wrote the guideline, who reviewed it, and who funded it. The best guidelines are specific about these matters. Guidelines may be funded by governments, charity organizations, health care funding insurance companies, or pharmaceutical companies. Regardless of how the guideline was funded, it is important to assess what the professional relationship of the writers and reviewers of the guideline is to the people who are providing funding. For example, even though the guideline may have been funded by a government agency (presumably with no vested interest other than effective and efficient health care), one or more writers or reviewers may be receiving grants from pharmaceutical companies for work other than guideline development. The best guidelines describe these relationships and assure that there is no conflict of interest.

Next, make sure the guideline describes how the evidence was collected. The search must be thorough, including the dates of the research evidence used in the guideline.

The manner in which the evidence is assessed and graded must be thoroughly described. If the "evidence" is "a consensus by a group of authorities," don't go any further. There may be other guidelines based more on good research than on the opinions of experts who may have a vested interest.

The best evidence comes from a systematic review of all the randomized controlled trials dealing with the treatment of the condition you are reviewing.[6] If there are only a few RCTs but they are well done and all agree with the others, this is also excellent evidence. The next best evidence is well-designed controlled trials without randomization. After this is evidence from well-designed cohort or case-control studies, preferably from more than one centre or research group.

Then there is evidence obtained from comparisons between times or places with or without the intervention.

Dramatic results in uncontrolled experiments (such as the results of treatment with penicillin in the 1940s) could also be included in this category.

If the only "evidence" is the opinion of respected authorities, based on clinical experience, descriptive studies or reports of expert committees, look for another guideline.

Producers of guidelines often develop codes to indicate the strength of the recommendation. For example, an "A" recommendation should be based on good evidence (RCTs) that the intervention be performed. A "B" recommendation should be based on cohort or case-controlled studies—"fair" evidence that the intervention be performed. A "C" recommendation means that there is "poor" evidence regarding the value or harm of the intervention, for example the PSA screening. A "D" recommendation suggests that there is fair evidence that the intervention *not* be performed—cohort or case-control studies showing the intervention not to be beneficial or in fact harmful. An "E" recommendation means that there is good evidence to support the recommendation that the intervention *not* be performed, for example, RCTs showing it not to be beneficial or even harmful.

Although the well-recognized evidence-based guideline producers may not use exactly the same system as outlined above, they do describe their methods of evaluating the evidence behind the recommendations and the systems used are similar.

If you do not have the time, interest, or patience to look for all the above details in determining whether a guideline is the right one for you, consider looking at guidelines which have been reviewed in the manner outlined in this chapter and summarized for easy application. The group that reviews, evaluates, and summarizes guidelines with which I am most familiar is the Guideline Advisory Committee, a joint committee of the Province of Ontario Ministry of Health and Long-term Care and the Ontario Medical Association. I am a member of the committee. Medical librarians carefully review the research literature regarding guidelines on a wide range of topics. When a condition such as hypertension is chosen, the most recent and applicable guidelines are sent to four different physician-reviewers (none of whom has any conflict of interest) who independently rate the guidelines using a scale of one to four for each of the qualities looked for in good guidelines. These reviews are then assessed a second time by the whole committee and the highest-rated guideline is then summarized and placed on the committee's website (www.gacguidelines.ca).

In the case scenario regarding hypertension, there is good evidence that treating high blood pressure with medications (when lifestyle changes like diet, exercise, smoking cessation are not sufficient) lowers the incidence of strokes by thirty-five to forty per cent, heart attacks by twenty-five per cent, and heart failure by fifty per cent.

Should you take the low-cost, generic medication prescribed by your physician, or a newer, more expensive product? The guideline selected by the Guideline Advisory Committee advises that your physician is right—there is good evidence from randomized controlled trials that the older, less expensive generic medication is very effective at controlling high blood pressure in many cases, and that the newer products need only be considered if the desired result is not obtained.[7] This approach is supported in a more recent guideline.[8]

Clinical practice guidelines, especially when there is disagreement between various CPGs, can present a challenge for the physician, and even more so for the patient.

If you as a patient have reviewed CPGs on a problem that affects you, and feel that you cannot assess which one of conflicting guidelines is based on better evidence, you should arrange a visit with your doctor. Let your doctor know that the objective of the visit is to go over the CPGs so that you can both decide which recommendations are best for you.

Here is a list of guidelines that are free to the general public. Those on the list have been chosen because they are up-to-date, evidence-based, and relatively easy to use.

1. American College of Physicians (ACP)
    Clinical Practice Guidelines:
    http://www.acponline.org/clinical/guidelines
2. British Columbia's Guidelines and Protocols
    Advisory Committee
    Clinical Practice Guidelines and Protocols in
    British Columbia:
    http://www.hlth.gov.bc.ca/msp/protoguides/index.
    html
3. Canadian Task Force on Preventive Health Care
    Systematic Reviews & Recommendations:
    http://www.ctfphc.org/

4. CMA Infobase Clinical Practice Guidelines:
   http://mdm.ca/cpgsnew/cpgs/index.asp

5. United States Department of Health & Human
   Services—Agency for Healthcare Research & Quality
   Evidence-based Practice Centers Evidence Reports:
   http://www.ahrq.gov/clinic/epcix.htm

6. Institute for Clinical Systems Improvement (ICSI)
   Health Care Guidelines:
   http://www.icsi.org/knowledge/browse_bydate.asp?
   CATID=:29

7. National Guideline Clearinghouse (NGC)
   Evidence-Based Clinical Practice Guidelines:
   http://www.guideline.gov/

8. Australian Government National Health and
   Medical Research Council Clinical Practice
   Guidelines:
   http://www.nhmrc.gov.au/publications/subjects/
   clinical.htm

9. National Institute for Health and Clinical
   Excellence (NICE) Guidance:
   http://www.nice.org.uk/page.aspx?o=cat.
   diseasearcas

10. New Zealand Guidelines Group
    Guidelines/Publications:
    http://www.nzgg.org.nz/index.cfm?fuseaction_10

11. Scottish Intercollegiate Guidelines Network
    Guidelines:
    http://www.sign.ac.uk/guidelines/published/
    index.html

12. ProdigyGuidance:
http://www.prodigy.nhs.uk/search/0/
clinical_practice_guidelines
13. National Electronic Library of Health (NeLH)
Guidelines Finder:
http://libraries.nelh.nhs.uk/guidelinesFinder

References:

1. "Committee to Advise the Public Health Service on Clinical Practice Guidelines, Institute of Medicine." Field, M.J., Lohr, K.N., editors. *Clinical practice guidelines: directions for a new program.* National Academy Press, Washington, 1990. p38

2. Fletcher, S.W., Fletcher, R.W. "Development of Clinical guidelines—Commentary." *The Lancet* 352, 1876, 1998

3. National Institutes of Health Consensus Development Panel. "National Institute of Health consensus development conference statement: breast cancer screening for women ages 40–49," Jan.21–23, 1997—Monographs National Cancer Institute, 22: vii–xviii, 1997

4. Eastman, P. "NCI adopts new mammography screening guidelines for women." *Journal of the National Cancer Institute*, 89: 8–10, 1997

5. Shekelle, P.G., Ortiz, E., Rhodes, S., et al. "Validity of the Agency for Healthcare Research and Quality Clinical Practice Guidelines: How Quickly Do Guidelines Become Outdated?" *JAMA*, 286: 1461–1467, 2001

6. *Evidence-Based Pediatrics*, Feldman, W., editor, B.C. Decker Inc. Hamilton, London, Saint Louis, 2000

7. "Canadian Hypertension Recommendations Working Group (2001)." *Canadian Journal of Cardiology.* 17(5): 535–38

8. "The Seventh Report of the Joint National Committee on Prevention, Detection, Evaluation, and Treatment of High Blood Pressure." *JAMA*, 289(19): 2560–72, 2003

CHAPTER 10

We Need More Evidence

Despite the growth of the evidence-based medicine movement, what I call "faith-based medicine" still prevails, in both developing (where the use of magic and shamans might be the only current option) and developed countries.

While the use of magic is more understandable in developing countries, what are the reasons for its prevalence as a form of or extension to traditional medicine within the developed world? On the one hand, it is possible that some patients have lost confidence in medical doctors and wish to make more of their health care decisions on their own, using information to which they have ever-increasing access. On the other hand, it is likely that many patients seek to augment their traditional treatments; again, this is based on information received through advertising or on the Internet. However, it is vital to distinguish between information and evidence. Information is defined as "knowledge acquired or derived; facts." In other words, if a health care provider (doctor, alternative medical provider, pharmaceutical company) informs you—in the media or on the Internet—that a treatment or product works, many patients accept the statement as fact, and use the product or procedure. The problem is that there may be no evidence that the treatment or product is either effective or safe. An even greater problem is that many patients a) do not think it is important to assess the evidence, and b) do not know how to assess the evidence.

In the developed world, science has led to many beneficial changes in our everyday lives and yet the culture of inquiry, data gathering, and evaluation, which forms the foundation of the best researchers' work, has not been passed down to people who need and use health care. Most patients still live in a faith-based as opposed to an evidence-based health care culture.

Cultural changes take time but are possible.

During the past fifty years, the developed world has seen a widespread growth in alternative health providers—homeopaths, naturopaths, herbalists, and others. Complementary and alternative medicine (CAM) is now used by more than forty per cent of the U.S. public. Herbal medicine use increased by almost four hundred per cent during the 1990s.[1]

In the U.S., total visits to CAM providers in 1997 exceeded by almost three hundred million the total visits to primary care physicians. The belief in these practitioners is, to some extent, age-related: only three in ten pre–baby boomers but seven in ten post–baby boomers report the use of at least one CAM therapy by the age of thirty-three.[2]

I stress CAM therapies because they are the best example of treatments not based on scientific evidence occupying the role that medical doctors played before effective preventive and treatment practices based on good evidence became available.

That some CAM therapies are completely unfounded is understood when one reviews the premises upon which their existence is based. For example, homeopathy is based on the concept that highly diluted traces of botanical, mineral, and other natural substances stimulate the body's self-healing abilities. Whereas it is entirely possible that botanical, mineral, and other natural substances may be beneficial, the foundation of homeopathy rests on the belief that the more dilute the substances, the more effective they are. The analogy is that if an adult dose of aspirin helps your headache, you would get even more relief if you took one hundredth of a baby dose or less.

Some would say that they still believe in homeopathy, even if medical doctors think it doesn't make sense. They argue that medical doctors are against homeopathy because if patients go to a homeopath instead of a physician, this would affect the physician's income. However, the evidence of the research published in the scientific literature supports doctors and not homeopaths. A recent review of placebo-controlled trials of homeopathy, published in *The Lancet*, showed "little evidence of effectiveness of any single homeopathic approach on any single clinical condition."[3]

Another CAM treatment, which makes no biologic sense, and yet is becoming more and more popular, is therapeutic touch. The therapist actually does not touch the patient, but moves his or her hands around the body in a flowing motion, a few inches away from the body. This is supposed to "work with the person's energy flow as a means of inducing relaxation and speed the healing process."[4]

In fact, a randomized controlled trial of therapeutic touch showed it to be no more effective than placebo.[5]

What about the other eighteen or so CAM therapies (like acupressure or aromatherapy)? The good news is that there are scientists in North America and the U.K. who are researching the effectiveness of these procedures so that we will hopefully soon know which, if any, do more good than harm. In an attempt to bring some consistency and a measure of scientific information to the public, the National Institute for Health (U.S.) has set up the National Center for Complementary and Alternative Medicine.

I mention harm because just as there are side effects that are known about traditional medical treatments, there are significant side effects of some of the CAM therapies. The problem is that whereas medical treatments, especially medications, are government regulated—what they are made of and the amount of medication in each pill or teaspoon—herbal and homeopathic treatments are poorly regulated. There are serious problems with the overall quality and safety of some of these products. In one study of ginseng products, the amount in the bottle of the presumed active ingredients compared to the amount on the label varied from twelve per cent to more than three hundred per cent! The recent death of a

Baltimore Orioles pitcher who took supplements containing ephedra has received a lot of attention. Another example of harm that may be caused by herbal medicine is cancer of the genitourinary system, associated with the Chinese herb Aristolochia fangchi. Although banned in Canada, Australia, and Germany, a recent report in the *New England Journal of Medicine* described its ready availability in capsule form in the United States. Other well-documented examples of harm associated with herbs include hepatitis and the herb germander, other liver problems related to comfrey, as well as kidney failure and convulsions related to yohimbe. Dietary supplements are also the cause of some concern as they too are unregulated. A recent U.S. survey revealed "widespread and potentially dangerous public ignorance of the regulation and labelling of vitamins, minerals, and food supplements." In that survey, most people believed that dietary supplements must be approved by a government agency, that producers of these substances cannot make claims about their effectiveness and safety unless there is good supporting evidence, and that the government requires that labels show potential dangers. Although this is true for pharmaceuticals, which are government regulated, it is *not* necessarily true for supplements.

In 2004, the Canadian government required that all "health products" be officially classified as drugs under the Natural Health Product Directorate. However, products that did not make "health" claims were categorized as foods, which are loosely regulated. Since then, of about 60,000 products available at health food stores only about 450 have been approved. There is pressure on the government to put all supplements in the food category so that the regulation would be much less than if they were in the drug category.[6]

Many health care consumers and providers believe that dietary supplements are not only beneficial but also that they must be safe because their contents are usually found in the foods we eat. For example, large doses of vitamin A, C, and E, as well as beta carotene, are widely used because of their so-called antioxidant effect. Some early studies suggested that these dietary supplements in large doses could prevent cancer of the gastrointestinal system. In fact, when all the studies were carefully and systematically reviewed (fourteen randomized controlled trials involving more than 170,000 patients), no protection against gastrointestinal cancer was found. Even worse, the mortality rate in the groups taking large doses of vitamins A, C, E, and beta carotene was *higher* than that in the groups taking placebos.[7]

In reviewing research involving any treatment, whether it is an accepted medication prescribed by a physician or a treatment prescribed by an alternative practitioner, it is important to know how the research was funded. For example, most of the research showing that glucosamine relieved joint pain in people with osteoarthritis was industry funded. When independently funded studies (studies funded by a university or a government agency as opposed to the company making the product) were conducted, they showed that patients receiving glucosamine were no better off than patients receiving placebo.[8]

Does the public really relate more to practitioners of CAM than to physicians, and if so, is it because CAM providers spend more time with patients, or relate better, or are more charismatic? Is it that a patient's level of education is a factor in his or her choice of a CAM provider of a physician? Are the two mutually exclusive—do some patients seek both CAM providers and physicians for the same ailment? How many patients believe, like Ivan Illich, in his 1975 book *Medical Nemesis*, that "the medical establishment has become a major threat to health"? Or, do more patients have greater expectations for their health, feeling perhaps that additional treatments will be beneficial? Many factors could influence the increase in visits to alternative practitioners, including whether certain groups (such as osteopaths, chiropractors, and those who practice acupuncture) are included in a nation's health care system.

However, despite the increasing use of CAM practitioners, the evidence suggests that most patients still relate to medical practitioners and are reasonably satisfied with the care they receive. In a recent survey, patients in Canada rated highly the access to family physicians and the quality of care provided. In another survey, ninety per cent of hospitalized patients rated the care provided by their physicians as excellent or good.

Although one study finds that CAM providers spend more time with patients than do physicians, this is certainly not always the case. In Beijing I saw long lineups of patients waiting to be diagnosed and treated by a CAM provider—a herbalist. The interaction took less than a minute with most of the time spent writing the herbal prescription.

There is a study that shows the educational status of CAM patients to be slightly higher than those who choose medical doctors only. I know people with PhDs who prefer homeopathy, so lack of formal education is not a major factor.

There is good evidence that, especially for patients with chronic conditions, both CAM providers and physicians are often involved. In some studies of patients attending medical practitioners for chronic conditions such as cancer or arthritis, more than fifty per cent also attend CAM practitioners.

Finally, although there are patients who share Illich's negative ideas about doctors and the health care they provide, like those parents who refuse to have their children immunized for fear of perceived complications such as autism, I believe that these individuals are in a minority.

In summary, most patients choose their health care providers (either CAM practitioners, medical doctors, or both) not because the practitioner employs approaches based on the best available evidence but rather because the patients have faith in their chosen practitioner and hope that he or she will help keep them well and/or make them healthy again. Given the bad news about Vioxx and other treatments early in the twenty-first century, it appears as though many patients are having serious questions as to whether that faith is well founded.

I hope that readers of this book will better understand the current state of events and will be armed with the approaches required to make the best decisions regarding their health care.

References:

[1] Verghese, A., *New York Times*, 12/8/02, from Medscape Primary Care.

[2] Ibid.

[3] Linde, K., Clausius, N., Ramirez, G., et al. "Are the clinical effects of homeopathy placebo effects? *A meta analysis* of placebo-controlled trials." *The Lancet*, 350:834–43, 1997

[4] Harden, B.L., and Harden, C.R. *Alternative Health Care—The Canadian Directory*, Noble Ages Publishing Ltd., 1997, p228

[5] Blankfield, R.P., Sulzmann, C., Fradley, L.G., et al. "Therapeutic touch in the treatment of carpal tunnel syndrome." *Journal of the American Board of Family Medicine*, Sept-Oct; 14(5):335–42, 2001

[6] Vasil, A., *Now Magazine*, June 2–8, 2005

[7] Bjelakovic, G., Nikolova, D., Simonetti, R.G., Gluud, C. "Antioxidant Supplements for Prevention of Gastrointestinal Cancers: a Systematic Review and Meta-analysis." *The Lancet*, Oct 2; 364(9441):1219–28, 2004

[8] McAlinden, T., Formica, M., La Valley, M., et al. "Effectiveness of Glucosamine for Symptoms of Knee Arthritis." *American Journal of Medicine,* Vol 117, Nov 1/04

CHAPTER 11

Summary and Conclusions

Throughout the centuries, patients saw their physicians as healers and believed that doctors could prevent disease, cure their illnesses, and alleviate their symptoms when cure was impossible. Science has become more and more the foundation of medical practice and physicians increasingly are recommending preventive and curative interventions that are evidence-based— interventions that have been shown in well-conducted research studies to do more good than harm. The public, however, continues to seek health care that has not been well researched.

There are a number of reasons why many patients are choosing unproven, unscientific measures in favour of or in addition to Western medicine. One is the media. As the media see it, "good news is no news." There is little media coverage of the reasons for the increasing lifespans of citizens, which is largely due to effective medical care when citizens have access to it. Medical errors, unpredicted side effects of widely used medicines, dramatic stories of "cures" caused by alternative practitioners, etc. are reported much more often. The media must recognize that selling ads and reaping profits, while important, are only one of their mandates; informing the public with accurate, relevant, and evidence-based information is equally if not more important.

Complementary and alternative medicine (CAM), consisting of over eighteen therapies—most of which have not been shown to do more good than harm—have become increasingly popular in the developed world. Well-proven preventive manoeuvres such as childhood immunizations are being avoided by many parents because of a belief that they are harmful, even though there is ample evidence that they do infinitely more good than harm.

Another reason for the increasing use of CAM therapies is cultural. Our education system is not turning out students who are taught to think for themselves, to ask questions, and to obtain the evidence necessary to answer their questions. "Science, magic, and religion," medical sociologists inform us, serve as the foundation of the relationships between doctors and patients. Our education systems must address a glaring lack of science in their curricula, starting in grade schools. The increasing use of CAM therapies that have no research support is a reflection that in the developed world, in the twenty-first century, magic is still part of our culture, proof that our schools are not graduating students who know how to obtain and evaluate evidence.

The pharmaceutical companies and their relationships with doctors are another reason for the public's lessening of confidence in the medical profession. High prices due to excessive profits, withholding information about important side effects, suppressing the publication in medical journals of negative results of drug trials, direct-to-consumer advertising causing patients to put pressure on doctors to prescribe expensive medicines when less expensive or no medication may lead to results that are just as good—all of these cause patients to doubt Western medicine. When drug companies pay for physicians to attend medical conferences, sometimes at luxurious resorts, these physicians are likelier to prescribe that company's products, even though other less expensive medications may be equally effective and safe.

Governments must also take some of the blame. In the U.S., Food and Drug Advisory panels have many scientists tied to private drug companies. This may allow new drugs to be put on the market before they have been shown to be more effective and/or safer than existing medications. Medical journals must be more attentive to the authors' potential conflicts of interest when reviewing research or review articles touting a particular drug or treatment.

A significant factor in the major improvements in the duration and quality of life in the past century has been preventive medicine. Immunizations have saved the lives of millions of children. Ideally, preventive manoeuvres should be studied by randomized controlled trials. This is the case for the commonly used childhood vaccines which have been shown to do far more good than harm. Poor science and media attention caused many parents to believe that some vaccines could lead to autism, leading many parents to refuse immunizations for their children: there is now good evidence that autism is in no way related to childhood vaccination. A number of cohort and case-control studies show that, if anything, there is a tendency for fewer autistic children to have had MMR than non-autistic children. Thus, in making decisions about any preventive intervention, people should assess whether well-designed RCTs have been done showing the manoeuvre to do more good than harm. If RCTs have not been done, there should be cohort or case-control studies showing that people who have had the preventive intervention are better off than those who have not.

Screening tests done on people without evidence of a disease should have been shown in RCTs to do more good than harm. Identifying the potential of developing a problem years after the test makes patients, their families, and their employers very anxious. Unless the test reveals with a high degree of accuracy that there is a real risk and unless there is something which can be done to reliably prevent the disease from developing, one should seriously question having the test done. The PSA test which screens for prostate cancer is an example of a test which has been widely promoted and taken up by doctors and patients before the results of RCTs are known. Breast self-examination is another screening procedure which was advocated and adopted by millions of women before the results of RCTs which showed no difference in mortality between women who regularly did BSE and those who did not.

False positive screening tests cause great anxiety and unnecessary surgery.

Screening tests should not be promoted until there is good evidence that the tests are accurate and precise and that early intervention is more beneficial than knowing about a potential problem is harmful.

The results of a RCT of PSA screening will be known by the year 2007.

Other examples of screening tests and how to assess whether they should be performed are described in Chapter 6. These include prenatal ultrasounds, Pap smears for cervical cancer, colonoscopy for colorectal cancer, and cholesterol screening.

Laboratory tests or x-rays are not always necessary for a correct diagnosis to be made. Studies have been done which show, for example, that in adults the diagnosis of strep throat can be made without the throat swab which proves that the bacteria streptococcus caused the sore throat. If an adult under forty-five years with a sore throat has a fever greater than 38°C (100.4°F), has tender glands in the neck, has no significant cough, and has swelling or pus on the tonsils, the likelihood of strep being the cause is so high that antibiotics could be given without the swab.

Similarly, until recently, doctors regularly did ankle x-rays to rule out a fracture in patients with sprained ankles. The Ottawa Ankle Rules, based on excellent studies in which all patients had x-rays as the gold standard are now used in many countries. A history of being able to bear weight, even with a limp, both at the time of the injury and when assessed by the doctor, when combined with the examination by the doctor, makes the likelihood of a fracture virtually zero. No fractures were found in many hundreds of patients with ankle sprains who met these criteria. Doctors who use the Ottawa Ankle Rules have been able to save significant amounts of money by reducing the number of ankle x-rays. In addition, many patients have to spend much less time in emergency rooms because they do not have to have ankle x-rays performed.

In addition to a number of tests being unnecessary to make a diagnosis, many tests are done in an attempt to understand why a particular illness occurred in a specific patient. Does the patient have an underlying abnormality which caused the illness? Could it be serious and lead to a worsening of the underlying problem? An example of this is x-ray tests of the kidneys, ureters, and bladder in children who have a bladder or kidney infection.

In these children urine tests are necessary to confirm that an infection in the genitourinary system is the cause of the symptoms. However, there is little evidence that for otherwise healthy children over two years old, x-rays of the kidneys, ureters, and bladder are beneficial. Should the infection recur, or should the child become quite ill with another urinary infection, x-rays may be necessary.

Doctors make diagnoses by taking a focused history, doing a physical examination, and, when necessary, doing the smallest number of lab tests needed to make a diagnosis. Tests should be compared with a gold standard to make sure that they are accurate. A good example of a gold standard is a biopsy or an autopsy where the problem can be seen under the microscope.

The electrocardiogram in patients suspected of having a heart attack has been validated by autopsies of patients who died of heart attacks.

In those few cases where the doctor suspects a heart attack but the EKG is not significantly abnormal, a blood test which shows that there has been heart muscle destruction will help make the diagnosis.

In addition to being compared to a gold standard, the studies regarding the value of a lab test should have been done on patients similar to the patient being seen. There should be good inter-observer reliability of the test—the same EKG shown to two different doctors should be interpreted in the same way. Also the definition of "abnormal" should be clear—most blood tests are scaled according to percentiles, where the top 2.5 per cent are considered high, or having a blood sugar suggesting the possibility of diabetes. The bottom 2.5 per cent of blood tests are considered low, with a blood hemoglobin suggesting anemia. Since anyone, including a healthy person, has a five per cent chance of having an abnormal test, these findings have to be placed in context with how the patient feels and what the doctor finds.

To determine prognosis, or the cause of a disease and the probability of recovery, the evidence should be based on follow-ups of patients like the one being considered, in terms of severity of the illness and the stage at discovery. Other factors like gender, age, and social class which may have an impact on the course of the disease should also be considered when reviewing the evidence on prognosis. In addition the follow-up should be long enough to get an accurate prognosis. As many patients as possible should be followed up for as long as possible in order to be sure about cure rates and mortality rates.

The benefits and risks associated with a treatment should be based on randomized controlled trials, whenever possible conducted in a double-blind manner. This means that neither the patient nor the researcher assessing the effect of the treatment should be aware of whether the new treatment, the standard treatment, or the placebo was taken. At the end of the study the researchers and patients should be informed about the grouping. The groups should be as similar as possible in factors which might affect the outcome, such as age, gender, severity of illness, and social class. The sample size should be large enough so that any outcome differences found are likely due to the treatment and not due to chance alone. Similarly the sample should be large enough so that if no differences are found in outcome this is because the new treatment was no better than the standard therapy or placebo, and not due to chance. The patients should be followed for long enough to be certain that any benefits found outweighed the risks of the treatment.

Finally, as many of the patients in the study as possible should be followed to the end of the research. Did patients not accounted for at the end not show up because they were cured, possibly on the placebo? Or were they found dead, possibly on the new treatment?

Clinical practice guidelines (CPGs) are being produced and promoted to assist physicians and patients in making decisions about appropriate health care. Not all physicians use them because CPGs developed by different groups come up with differing recommendations. CPGs written by groups without a financial conflict of interest—not funded by pharmaceutical or other businesses—are the first to be looked at. The CPG should be up-to-date and should be developed using sound evidence—the best CPGs are systematic reviews of randomized controlled trials. Next on the list should be evidence of well-designed controlled trials without randomization, followed by good cohort or case-control studies. Dramatic evidence from comparisons between times or places with or without the intervention (penicillin in the 1940s) can also be helpful. The least valuable evidence in a CPG is based on the opinions of respected authorities based on their clinical experience or consensus from committees.

A new development is the Ontario Guideline Advisory Committee, which is government funded. Its mandate is to review and evaluate guidelines, to summarize and disseminate the best guidelines to health care workers, and to promote their use.

Although I have described in detail some of the pitfalls that still exist in the health care received by some patients, the good news is that evidence-based medicine is spreading rapidly throughout the developed world. In addition, medical schools are stressing more and more the importance of doctor-patient communication, empathy, integrity and competence. In fact, medical societies in the U.S., Canada, and Europe have accepted a document entitled The Physician's Charter. This charter essentially commits physicians to many of the key points stressed in this book—professional competence, largely based on evidence-based medicine, honesty, confidentiality, access to care, avoiding conflict of interest, and commitment to improving medicine by facilitating good research.

Many medical schools are teaching courses in complementary and alternative medicine and promoting research in this area.

The future looks good. When health care providers and their patients are armed with the best evidence, they can together make the right decisions about health care.

Index